HEALTH AND RESILIENCE

HEALTH AND RESILIENCE

Edited by
TADEUSZ MARIAN OSTROWSKI
IWONA SIKORSKA

JAGIELLONIAN UNIVERSITY PRESS

The publication of this volume was supported by The Faculty of Applied Psychology of the Jagiellonian University.

REVIEWER
prof. dr hab. Nina Ogińska-Bulik

COVER DESIGN
Jadwiga Burek

ISBN 978-83-233-3625-9

www.wuj.pl

Jagiellonian University Press
Editorial Offices: Michałowskiego St. 9/2, 31-126 Kraków
Phone: 12-631-18-81, 12-631-18-82, fax 12-631-18-83
Sales: Phone 12-631-01-97, Phone/Fax 12-631-01-98
Mobile: 506-006-674, e-mail: sprzedaz@wuj.pl
Bank account: PEKAO SA, no. 80 1240 4722 1111 0000 4856 3325

TABLE OF CONTENTS

Introduction 7

I. SOCIAL AND METHODOLOGICAL CONTECTS OF RESILIENCE

Tadeusz Marian Ostrowski
Resilience in the light of research and theoretical reflection 13

Konrad Banicki
Naturalism, normativism and Havi Carel's phenomenological approach
to health and illness 25

Krzysztof Gerc
Testing the sense of identity in people with highly functioning autism
as theory-methodological problem 39

Urszula Tokarska
"The beneficial life stories." Health and mental resilience from
the narrative perspective 57

II. RESILIENCE IN DEVELOPMENT

Iwona Sikorska
Theoretical models of resilience and resilience measurement tools
in children and young people 85

Bogusława Piasecka, Krzysztof Gerc, Iwona Sikorska
Siblings – a retrospective analysis of deidentification processes 101

Klaus Fröhlich-Gildhoff, Maike Rönnau-Böse
Empower children! The promotion of resilience in early childhood
institutions (kindergarten) and primary schools 117

III. RESILIENCE AND DISEASE

Władysława Pilecka
Resilience as a chance of developmental success for a child
with a chronic illness 141

Wojciech Otrębski, Barbara Czuba
Coping with stress amongst families with children suffering from chronic
psychosomatic diseases – recommendations for psychoprophylactic
actions 157

6

Izabella Januszewska, Stanisława Steuden
Styles of coping with negative emotions and stress in patients
with hypertension 169

Krzysztof Gerc, Marta Jurek
Family life dimensions and self-assessment of adolescents and young
adults using psychoactive substances – the comparative study 193

List of Authors 211

INTRODUCTION

The concept of resilience belongs to the category of positive terms, which are very inspiring to theoretical reflection and empirical studies in psychology. It has importance for the overall psychological theory and, in particular, for the theory of emotions and motivation, personality theory and the researches on psychological stress. The concept, furthermore, can be significantly referred to existential, social, and ecological psychology. Resilience is not only one of the basic categories in positive psychology, but also the one that has applications to psychology of development, psychology of education, family psychology as well as to health psychology and psycho-neuro-immunology. The significance of this concept for clinical and rehabilitation psychology can finally be added. The broadness of the area in which research on resilience is conducted, depicts very well the importance of this concept and its versatility.

The authors of the monography faced questions about the determinants of resilience, its mechanisms and consequences. Monography consists of three parts, namely I. Social and methodological contexts of resilience, II. Resilience in development, III. Resilience and disease.

The first one focuses on social and methodological contexts of resilience. There are four chapters in this part, all of them consider mainly theoretical questions connected with health, illness, healing, recover and well-being in the mental and bodily field.

The publication begins from the theoretical chapter, written by Tadeusz M. Ostrowski, which contains an overview of the basic conceptualization of resilience and trends of research in the latter, regarding the determinants of resistance, its mechanisms as well as developmental and health-related consequences. The author puts the term of resilience in the context of research on emotions, coping with stress and post-traumatic growth. In accordance with his interests, furthermore, he develops the direction of research, connected with the existential conditions of resilience.

The second chapter written by Konrad Banicki, in turn, addresses the most general metatheoretial and conceptual issues connected with the notion of health and its counterparts such as the concepts of illness and disease. Its main part refers to the phenomenological account of illness as provided by the British philosopher Havi Carel. This first-person perspective, importantly, is discussed against the background of two third-person approaches, which are currently dominant in the philosophy of medicine. The medical naturalism formulated by Christopher Boorse as well as the normativist position developed by Lennart Nordenfelt are accordingly analyzed.

The main issue in the Krzysztof Gerc's article is sense of identity in people with highly functioning autism. The concept of identity containing the following triad: competence, conception and condition by Lech Witkowski is a theoretical base for author's considerations. For the purposes of identity diagnostics in people with Asperger Syndrom or Highly Functioning Autism it is postulated to apply the narrative approach. Gerc proposes a hypothetical model of mutual interactions between social competence, intelligence, interests and isolated social skills, and self-assessment, as well as their connection to the process of identity formation.

Urszula Tokarska explores in her article mental health and resilience in the narrative dimension. She presents the beneficial life stories, which show and promote a healthy and well-functioning adult personality in its polyphonic structure. The narrative promotion of mental health and resilience opens up a chance for its recipients to transcend the automatic and unconscious understanding of life events. The concept of the narrative promotion of mental health and resilience emerges as an interesting area to develop in a therapeutic practice and in existential counselling.

The second monograph's part is devoted to resilience in development. The presented studies disscuses recognizing and measurement of resilience phenomenon in children, promoting programs for children and role of family in the resilience forming processes.

The article by Iwona Sikorska presents in the synthetic way a summary of the main theoretical models of resilience and chosen resilience measurement tools in children and young people. Resilience treated as an developmental outcome, as a process and as personal assets are discussed in the paper. A chosen example of measurement instrument was given to each presented theoretical proposal: Kidscreen, The Healthy Kids Survey, DECA, DESSA and Resilience Scale SPP 18.

The next article by Bogusława Piasecka, Krzysztof Gerc and Iwona Sikorska is devoted the family relations, especially sibling's contact. On the theoretical background of Schachter's concept and Toman's theory of family constellations the authors follow up the connections between birth order and personality traits. The aim of interview analysis is answer to research question how does deidentification process proceed between sibling.

The last paper in this part is dedicated to the third wave in the resilience research-application of knowledge in the field in form of prevention, intervention and creating a protective system. Klaus Froehlich-Gildhoff and Maike Roennau-Boese present the promotion of resilience in early childhood institutions (kindergarten) and primary schools. The intervention programme "Empowering Children!" described by authors addresses early childhood institutions situated in areas with a high level of diversity (e.g. high percentage of immigrant families, high poverty levels, etc., and aims to empower them in the work with children, parents and teachers.

The third part of monograph contains four articles connected with various aspects of "health in disease."

Władysława Pilecka discusses resilience as a developmental chance for a child with a chronic illness. The author describes six aspects of well-being according to positive psychology in chronic ill children: self-acceptance, life purpose, personal growth, control over the environment, positive relations with others and autonomy. Pilecka concludes her consideration with assumption that the constant process of becoming a mature and well-functioning person in children and youth with chronic somatic disease means every day battling against the demands and limitations. In the subject perspective, this process proceeds from an inevitable dependence on others towards a more and more dynamic self-creation.

Chronic ill children and their families are the focus topic in the article by Wojciech Otrębski and Barbara Czuba. The authors propose some guidelines for psycho-prophylactic actions promoting coping with stress amongst families with children suffering from chronic psychosomatic diseases. It is necessary to raise the level of social awareness concerning allergies and their prevention and better knowledge the process of how parents with chronically, psychosomatically sick children, cope with stress.

Izabella Januszewska and Stanisława Steuden tackle the subject of negative emotions and stress in patients with hypertension. Their comparative study presents styles of coping used by healthy individuals and used by people suffering from hypertension. The results suggest that people with hypertension show more intense use of emotional forms of coping with defensive avoiding-escaping behaviour and present much lower degree than healthy people operate in a cooperative style, so that they might receive support from people in their social environment.

Krzysztof Gerc and Marta Jurek present results of the comparative study with adolescents and young adults using psychoactive substances. Researched variables were family life dimensions and self-assessment of participants. Adolescents and young adults perceive their family functioning in terms of unpredictability of behaviour, lack of clarity of rules, organisational chaos, less intense bonds. It has been proved that individuals using psychoactive substances in research group show bigger difficulties in defining their own identity; they more often missed acceptance for themselves in their families and act against their own believes striving for presenting themselves as independent and non-conformists.

This publication is a collection of articles dealing with a topic of resilience looked at from many various perspectives. The authors present either quantitative approach to the psychological research (Gerc, Jurek, Januszewska, Froehlich-Gildhof, Roennau-Boese) or qualitative (Tokarska, Piasecka, Gerc, Sikorska).

Many authors discuss theoretic models, mechanisms and phenomena connected with health and resilience, and present overview of the body of literature in the field (Ostrowski, Banicki, Sikorska, Pilecka, Otrębski, Czuba).

While expressing our gratitude to all the authors for their engagement in this monograph's preparation, we hope that our mutual effort will have some impact on discussion on health, well-being and personal growth despite adversities. We believe that resilience research and discussion will develop successfully in our country and will enable to create preventive and promoting programs for children, youth and risk group in the community.

Editors

I. SOCIAL AND METHODOLOGICAL CONTECTS OF RESILIENCE

Tadeusz Marian Ostrowski
Jagiellonian University
The Institute of Applied Psychology

RESILIENCE IN THE LIGHT OF RESEARCH AND THEORETICAL REFLECTION

Abstract

Resilience has been characterized in the paperf from the perspective of a theoretical point of view and in the light of the results of empirical research. Two terms are used in the literature: *resiliency*, as a dispositional trait of personality and *resilience*, as the transactional process of relation between individual and environment and as the process of coping behaviour. The first meaning of the term is more emphasised in the paper. Psychological resiliency is discussed in the context of emotional and cognitive mechanisms. The next part of the article is devoted to determinants of resiliency from cognitive, social and existential point of view. Development and health implications of resiliency are discussed at the end of this paper.

Key words: resiliency, resilience, personality, coping, emotions, spirituality, religiosity, health

Resilience belongs to the positive psychological categories, which were established in order to clarify why the individual does not break down in the face of difficulties. The term comes from the 1950s, and its current popularity is connected with development of positive psychology and health psychology. Two similar terms used in the literature should be distinguished: *resiliency* as a dispositional trait of personality and *resilience* as the transactional process of relation between individual and environment and as the process of coping behaviour. The first meaning of the term is more emphasised in this paper.

It can be said that conceptof resiliency has salutogenic[1] meaning. In accordance to the intention of Antonovsky (1987), the essence of the salutogenic approach is the identification of personal dispositions, processes and mechanisms

---

[1] *Salus* (Latin) – health.

that make the man maintains health, despite a confrontation with serious stressful events. Besides it, mental resilience is a concept focused on the process in the same meaning as health and disease in salutogenic approach. Resilience is revealed in the act of "rising from the fall" after a difficult stressful event. The sooner individual goes out from a phase of mental trauma and return to normal functioning, the more one reveals the resilience.

Heszen and Sęk (2007, p. 173) define resilience as: "a conjunction of effective skills for coping with a large stress, which involve flexible, creative dealing with adversity; the main role is played here by the ability to *bounce-back* from negative experiences and the capacity to induce positive emotions."

The opposite of resiliency is vulnerability, susceptibility, sensitivity to stressors. To the category of opposite sense can be also include *Personality type D*. This construct will be discussed below.

Theoretical approach to resilience

Resilience is conceptualized in different ways. Most often one can find three approaches:

1. Resiliency as a feature of personality. In this aspect it is treated as a disposition to wrestling with life difficulties. It can be classified as mental health resources. Thus, like personality trait, it is conditioned on both sides: inheritance, mainly temperament characteristics and, on the other hand, influences of the environment. Such understanding of resiliency has been popularised in Poland by Ogińska-Bulik and Juczyński, who have published a number of research which have been carried out on the basis of this term (Ogińska-Bulik, Juczyński, 2010; Ogińska-Bulik, 2010, 2010b, 2011, 2011a). The authors used the questionnaire, developed by themselves, titled: *Resiliency Measurement Scale* SPP-25, and in versions for children and adolescents SPP-18 (Ogińska-Bulik, Juczyński, 2008; 2011).

2. Resilience in terms of transactional paradigm. In this context the resilience is treated as a transaction between the individual and the environment. Heszen and Sęk (2007) strongly emphasize the transactional nature of the resilience. It reveals a transaction between the individual and the situation in the stressful situation. Resilience in this approach does not depend so entirely on individual resources, but also on the properties of the stressful event and its context: social, cultural and ecological.

3. Resilience as an important mechanism in the process of coping. Transactional approach directly moves the issue of resilience into the area of research of coping with stress, especially with one's disease or disease or loss of close persons. The emotional resources, such as a tendency to generating positive emotions and skills of cognitive work with the difficult past (reappraisal)

increase the effectiveness of the resilience. The ability to concentrate on the task, high formal and emotional intelligence, and the variety of coping strategies are important conditions of resilience. On the other hand rumination and blaming others belongs to the strategies lower resilience.

The author of this paper in his research is using the term resiliency understood as the personality trait, which involves using the method of Ogińska-Bulik and Juczyński SPP-25 (2008). The understanding of resilience as a process is very inspirational, but it causes serious methodological problems.

Psychological mechanisms of resilience

In the literature psychological resilience mechanisms are divided into two groups: individual and social. The group of personal mechanism includes:
1. Emotional and even physical detachment from the situation of difficult, traumatic experience.
2. Generating of positive emotions, or rather their co-generating, next to the negative emotions associated with a difficult experience. The cognitive mechanisms of stressful event's development are following:
   (a) Davis, Nolen-Hoeksema and Larson (1998) wrote about changing of perception in stressful situation to find its positive aspects. This is a cognitive mechanism of reevaluating – *benefit finding*.
   (b) The same authors identified mechanism of finding meaning in a difficult experience through its place in a natural sequence of human life – *sense making*. There is some similarity to accepting of suffer – „attitude over the suffering," which Frankl described as *the attitudinal values* (1984, 2006).
   (c) Folkman and Moskowitz (2000) stated that occurrence of positive emotions are connected with a task-oriented coping style (*problem-focused coping*), moreoverwith the application of the strategy of positive reevaluation (*positive reappraisal*) and giving positive meaning to ordinary events (*infusing ordinary events with positive meaning*).
   (d) Fredrickson (1998, 2001) underlined that positive emotions are the basis of immunity. In her *the broaden-and-build theory of positive emotions*, author notes that both kinds of emotions – negative and positive, occur in response to the stress. Function of the negative emotions is to narrow one's mind to focus on the way to invade the obstacle, or to flee before it. In contrast to negative emotions, positive emotions (e.g., job satisfaction) expand one's mind functions that allow seeing the new aspects of the difficult situation, and also new ways of action, different from the existing. Broadening the area of perception and action builds individual physical, psychological and social resources.

(e) Tugade and Fredrickson (2004) cites research showing that resisted people develop their positive emotionality by generating positive emotions, using such strategies as sense of humour, relaxation techniques and positive thinking.

3. Another mechanism is a consistent realization of the goals, despite the subjective and situational difficulties, in conjunction with plastic, adapted to the situation strategies. A change of goals is told as an expression of resilience. However, the preservation of goal and changing the strategies can be treated as indicator of the resilience.

4. Cognitive mechanisms of developing difficult experiences are associated with abundant internal narration (internal dialogue). The rich, well-structured narration is a sign of cognitive transformation of event in time's dimension of past and present.

Turning to social mechanisms, it should be pointed out that this kind of mechanisms is related mainly to the creation of social support's network and to skills of using the social resources to supplement and multiplying the resilience (Sęk, Cieślak, 2004).

Resilience has also consequences at the level of the physiology. Negative emotions in a situation of stress cause arousal response to physiological and hormonal system in the fight-or-flight reaction. The resilient individuals are prone to generate also positive, not only negative emotions. On the other hand, the stimulation of the cardiovascular system after experiencing stressful event returns faster to the standard state in the case of resistant persons. In opinion of Fredrickson and Levenson (1998), emotional disposition to positive emotions can be used as an explanation of physiological evidences. This means that psychic mechanism for *bounce-back* has its component on the physiological level.

Determinants of resilience

Determinants of resilience are psychological and social in nature. One and the other areconsidered on different levels of generality.

Existential determinants of resilience include philosophy of life, beliefs, spirituality and religiosity. Peres, Moreira-Almeida, Nasello and Koenig (2007) cited the American data (Vieweget et al., 2006), which showed that the occurrence of traumatic events which were so serious, they could cause PTSD, is estimated at 50–90% of the population, while the diagnosis of PTSD did not exceed 8%. This difference authors explain by resilience, which causes that not always after the trauma comes to serious disorders. There is a question about the determinants of such resilience. The authors concluded that there are many considerations. They paid attention to religious coping, which turned out to be a popular strategy to cope with the trauma. After terrorist attack on the towers of the World Trade Center in New York City on September 11, 2001 the Americans coped with the trauma mostly by the conversation – 98%. The prayer and spiritual experiences were on the second place – 90% (Schuster et al., 2001).

Searching for explanations of the differences in reaction to trauma, Peres, Moreira-Almeida, Nasello, and Koenig (2007) stated that memories of trauma in people reacting in the form of PTSD are non-verbal in nature, because these people have difficulty in synthetic narration of traumatic event and assimilation of those experience to memory through a coherent narration. In opposition to them, the persons, which have not responded to the trauma by PTSD, express their memories in the form of a narration that is much more complete, internal structured, logical. Such characteristics of the narration that is reveals coping with trauma, which can be interpreted as a manifestation of resilience. Peres et al. (2007) paid attention to the results of the research with the use of neuro-imaging of the brain, explaining the cerebral mechanism for these differences. In a test group that reacted in the form of PTSD on trauma, authors of researches found reduced hippocampal activity, whose function is integration of a new event with individual cognitive map of experience. The authors confirmed synthetic, assessing and integrating role of the hippocampus in the formatting of cognitive map, included individual oneself and the environment. This weakness of this function of hippocampus is visible in fragmentary narration, which is characteristic for persons, which responded to trauma in the form of PTSD.

The spirituality is mentioned in literature as a predictor of resilience. This is the concept defined very differently in the social sciences (Ostrowski, 2010). In accordance to the theory of Hay (2007), spirituality is an innate psychic dimension. It has nature of a relational consciousness. Spirituality reveals, how Sperry wrote (2001), in early childhood as self-awareness. Then it gradually develops as a need to find meaning of action and capacity to transcendence, which is understood as going beyond one's own self into the world of values.

Kim and Esquivel (2011) stated, on the basis of a review of the research, that religiosity is mentioned in the literature as a second, independent predictor of mental resilience, next to the spirituality. The authors remarks, however, that these two concepts are defined in different paradigms. Spirituality is related to inner life of individual. The researchers locate this term in phenomenological-existential paradigm. They often accentuate its innate nature and biological determinants (Hay, 2007). On the other hand, religiosity is a kind of social activity, with cultural determination (socio-cultural paradigm). Many ideas of the authors concerning the meaning of both terms often overlap, but research should maintain their distinctness.

Crawford, Wright and Masten (2006) in a work on the importance of spirituality as a factor developing mental immunity of children and adolescents, mentioned four mechanisms, which are consequences of spirituality, namely: building interpersonal close ties, openness to social support in various forms, interiorization of standards and moral values and stimulation of human development. It should be told, that for a person who trusts in God, sources of social support include both the support from the social environment and the support from a supernatural, sacred area. Religiosity is most often cited as a positive predictor of resilience, but the authors indicate the possibility of the reverse relation. It may happen that religiosity reduces resilience, when strongly outweigh the sense of sinfulness, that isfavouredby image of God as a severe judge, rather than as a merciful father (Pargament, 1997).

The importance of spirituality as a predictor of resilience has been confirmed by Werner (1996) in her longitudinal, lasting more than 40 years research of 698 children from the Hawaiian Islands. The development of children was charged from the side of genetic predisposition and environmental circumstances. They grew up in conditions of poverty and a lack of healthy family relationships. Most of them, as expected, had suffered mental and physical impairment. As adults they had problems with the maintenance of the stability of their own family. However, one-third of children, despite the difficult conditions developed properly, realized social functions in a normal way. The factor which determines their resilience was, *inter alia*, spirituality, measured in this case as a form of religiosity and belonging to the Church. Of paramount importance was social support from the significant persons, such as parents, relatives, guardians or teachers. In the light of these results, it can be said that Werner has formed a question not only what caused the ontogenetic development disorders, but mainly what determined the fact that despite the pathogenic conditions for the development, children developed normally?

There is a similarity between Werner (1996) research and the theory of coherence, developed by Antonovsky (1987, 1991). The theory of coherence was mentioned in the first part of this article. According to this theory, the important determinant of resilience is the coherence with the world. Antonovsky has stated this regularity, as a result of the study, conducted in Israel. He examined the psychological functioning and mental health of women in menopause. As expected, the women, who were imprisoned in Nazi concentration camps as young girls, in a majority, tolerated menopausal period worse, compared to women, which were not in the camp. In the group of women who survived the camp, good health enjoyed just 29%, and in comparative group 51%. Attention of author caught the 29% of the women, former prisoners of concentration camps, who have enjoyed good health, in spite of very difficult past, the menopause and mature age. To explain the differences, Antonovsky created neologism *salutogenesis*. According to the theory, salutogenesis is the mechanism which determines the health, in opposition to the *pathogenesis* – set of causes of a disease. Antonovsky stated that in the mechanism of salutogenesis, high sense of coherence with the world, reflected in three aspects: *comprehensibility* – the belief that the world is understandable, *meaningfulness* – the world and human life have a sense, and *manageability* – there is possible to act on the world with success, was important. Such defined coherence determines the resilience in the light of the empirical results (Eriksson, Lindstrom, 2006). Antonovsky's research had the same theme as Werner: finding answer to the question what cause health despite the dynamic action of pathogenic factors. Question about mechanisms of health Antonovsky called salutogenic, as opposed to identifying the causes of disorder, which he described as a pathogenic question.

The problem of personality as a determinant of resiliency is brought up in the research of Fredrickson and Tugade (2003). They demonstrated that individuals with high scores on the *Ego-Resilience Scale* are characterized by Extroversion, low Neuroticism and high score on a Scale of Openness[2]. It should be depicted that in the dimensions of personality in Eysenck's theory, "resilient" score are located in the quarter of extroversion-neuroticism in opposition to persons with Type D personality, with negative emotionality, who are placed in the quarter of introversion-neuroticism. Individual with type D personality is prone to be worry, and to control of emotional expression, in order to avoid social danger. Hence there is the term "personality-prone-to-stress." Therefore, the Type D personality is contrasted to hardy personality (Kupper et al., 2013).

The hardy personality is an idea, developed by Kobasa (1983), which is connected to the problem of resilience. In the light of empirical evidences the author stated that the *hardy personality* is a construct with three components: *Commitment* – there is important belief in the meaning of actions, *Challenge* – connected with high self-efficacy and *Control* – sense of internal control in contradistinction to external control. It is worth mentioning that the hardness is associated with tenacity, hardy skills of fighting, to not surrender; while resilience means dealing with strategies flexible, up to the development of the situation, and a quick exit from the crisis.

An important determinant of resilience is the emotional intelligence, defined as the ability to differentiate one's own emotions and to recognize emotions of other people. This kind of intelligence is responsible for adequate using of emotions and interpersonal contact in the process of coping with difficulties (Salovey, Mayer, 1989–1990). Emotional intelligence is expressed, *inter alia*, as the ability to gather knowledge about one's own emotions, on the basis of life experience. Fredrickson (1998) underlined that this form of intelligence is associated with intuitive ability to respond in stress with positive emotions. This is typical for resistant persons. The positive emotions allow one to increase the resources of resilience in coping with stress.

Social determinants of resilience are connected with the size, availability and adequacy of social support, especially from the side of peer and family. It is important for individual to have the ability to establish the satisfactory emotional ties. They develop an individual social support network (Sęk, Cieślak, 2004).

---

[2] The authors chose three scales: Extroversion, Neuroticism and Openness from *NEO Five-Factor Inventory* (NEO-FFI).

The consequences of resiliency connected with development and health

Resiliency as the individual disposition has varied positive correlates with other processes that reveal themselves during life of the individual. These include the ability to reduce negative emotions in reaction to stress (anxiety, sadness, despair, resignation, anger), with simultaneous predominance of positive emotions. Fredrickson told about it in her, mentioned above *the broaden-and-build theory of positive emotions* (2001). The author presents results of research that high-resilient persons have optimistic attitude to the future and they are able to generate more positive emotions, compared with low-resilient. Remarkable are the results of the research in the group of students, carried out before the terrorist attack on the World Trade Center in New York City on September 11, 2001 and repeated about 3 weeks after the attack. Fredrickson and Tugade stated (2003), that the resilience is significantly correlated with six positive emotions out of ten, such as: interest, satisfaction, joy, hope, sexual desire and pride. In case of negative emotions, a significant negative correlation was only with two: anger and sorrow. The authors find that experiencing positive emotions helps greater resilience, which then increases the willingness to experience positive emotions and thus it starts the mechanism of positive feedback. This mechanism is the basis of the deal, which essence is the using of a wide range of strategies, adequately to the development of the situation, combined with the readiness to be flexible towards changes of situation (Fredrickson, Joiner, 2002).

Resilience promotes the posttraumatic growth. This conclusion revealed in the above mentioned investigation. Students after the terrorist attack unveiled a higher level of hope, satisfaction with life and optimism than before attack (Fredrickson, Tugade, 2003). Discussing these results Ogińska-Bulik and Juczyński (2008), they emphasized that resilience is a predictor of positive emotions after the crisis. High-resilient students after terrorist attack experienced less depression than sensitive students. Resilience plays a role of a buffer between stress and emotional response.

Returning to the issue of posttraumatic growth, the complexity of the relationship between the resiliency and the rise of growth should be noted. Ogińska-Bulik has revealed that the resilience is a good predictor of personal growth, but not the only one. Very important is the spirituality (Felcyn-Koczewska, Ogińska-Bulik, 2011; Ogińsk-Bulik, 2010a, 2013).

Interesting are the test results, indicating a positive correlation between the resilience and the state of health on psychic and physical level (Chanduszko-Salska, Ogińska-Bulik, 2011). Health is positively determined by *flourishing*. According to Fredrickson, this term means functioning onthe optimal level for the individual. The *flourishing* manifested by a sense of happiness, life satisfaction, personal growth and high level of resilience (Tugade, Fredrickson, Barrett, 2004).

Many studies confirm the relationship between the state of health and resilience, intermediated by spirituality and religiosity (Werner, 1996; Pargament, 1997), by a sense of meaning of life (Frankl, 1984, 2006), by sense of coherence (Antonovsky, 1987, 1991), and by positive attitudes towards people (Van Dyke, Elias, 2007).

In conclusion, it should be noted that resilience is an interdisciplinary category, of a great significance, could be treated as a source of inspiration of psychological theory and empirical research, but also used for practical applications in psychotherapy and crisis intervention, as well as in health promotion and prevention.

References

Antonovsky, A. (1987). *Unraveling The Mystery of Health – How People Manage Stress and Stay Well.* San Francisco: Jossey-Bass Publishers.

Antonovsky, A. (1991). *The Structural Sources of Salutogenic Strengths.* [In:] C.L. Cooper, R. Payne (Eds.). *Individual Differences: Personallity and Stress* (67–104). New York: Wiley.

Chanduszko-Salska, J., Ogińska-Bulik, N. (2011). *Prężność a ryzyko uzależnienia od jedzenia.* [W:] L. Golińska, E. Bielawska-Batorowicz (red.). *Rodzina i praca w warunkach kryzysu* (499–510). Łódź: Wyd. UŁ.

Crawford, E., Wright, M., Masten, A.S. (2006). *Resilience and spirituality in youth.* [In:] E.C. Roehlkepartain, P.E., King, L. Wagener., P.L. Benson (Eds.). *The handbook of spiritual development in childhood and adolescence* (355–370). Thousand Oaks, CA: Sage.

Davis, Ch.G., Nolen-Hoeksema, S., Larson, J. (1998). Making Sense of Loss and Benefiting From the Experience: Two Construals of Meaning. *Journal of Personality and Social Psychology*, 75(2), 561–574.

Felcyn-Koczewska, M., Ogińska-Bulik, N. (2011). *Rola prężności w rozwoju potraumatycznym osób w żałobie.* [W:] L. Golińska, E. Bielawska-Batorowicz (red.). *Rodzina i praca w warunkach kryzysu* (511–524). Łódź: Wyd. UŁ.

Folkman, S., Moskowitz, J.T. (2000). Positive affect and the other side of coping. *American Psychologist*, 55, 647–654.

Frankl, V.E. (1950). *Homo patiens. Versucheiner Pathodizee.* Wien: Franz Deuticke.

Frankl, V.E. (2006). *Man's search for meaning. An Introduction to Logotherapy.* Boston, MA: Beacon Press.

Fredrickson, B.L. (1998). What good are positive emotions? *Review of General Psychology: Special Issue: New Directions in Research on Emotion*, 2, 300–319.

Fredrickson, B.L. (2001). The role of positive emotions in positive psychology: The broaden-and-build theory of positive emotions. *American Psychologist*, 56, 218–226.

Fredrickson, B.L., Joiner, T. (2002). Positive emotions trigger upward spirals toward emotional well-being. *Psychological Science*, 13, 172–175.

22

Fredrickson, B.L., Levenson, R.W. (1998). Positive emotions speed recovery from the cardiovascular sequelae of negative emotions. *Cognition and Emotion*, 12, 191–220.

Fredrickson, B., Tugade, M., Waugh, Ch., Larkin, G. (2003). What good are positive emotions in crises? A prospective study of resilience and emotions following the terrorist attacks on the united states on September 11th, 2001. *Journal of Personality and Social Psychology*, 84, 365–376.

Hay, D. (2007). *The Biology of the Human Spirit*. Philadelphia: Templeton.

Heszen, I., Sęk, H. (red.). (2007). *Psychologia zdrowia*. Warszawa: Wydawnictwo Naukowe PWN.

Kim, S., Esquivel, G.B. (2011). Adolescent spirituality and resilience: theory, research, and educational practices. *Psychology in the Schools*, 48, 755–765.

Kobasa, S.C.O., Puccetti, M.C. (1983). Personality and social resources in stress resistance. *Journal of Personality and Social Psychology*, 45, 839–850.

Kupper, N., Pedersen, S., Höfer, S., Saner, H., Oldridge, N., Denollet, J. (2013). Cross-cultural analysis of Type D (distressed) personality in 6222 patients with ischemic heart disease: A study from the International HeartQoL Project. *International Journal Of Cardiology* [serial online], 166(2), 327–333.

Ogińska-Bulik, N. (2010). *Szkoła jako środowisko kształtowania psychologicznych zasobów jednostki chroniących przed podejmowaniem zachowań ryzykownych – rola prężności*. [W:] D. Bilski (red.). *Szkoła jako środowisko edukacji zdrowotnej* (21–34). Łódź: Wydawnictwo WSEZiNS.

Ogińska-Bulik, N. (2010a). Potraumatyczny rozwój w chorobie nowotworowej – rola prężności. *Polskie Forum Psychologiczne*, 15(2), 125–139.

Ogińska-Bulik, N. (2010b). Prężność a jakość życia młodzieży. *Psychologia Jakości Życia*, 1, 233–247.

Ogińska-Bulik, N. (2011). Rola prężności w zapobieganiu negatywnym skutkom stresu zawodowego. [W:] L. Golińska, E. Bielawska-Batorowicz (red.). *Rodzina i praca w warunkach kryzysu* (485–498). Łódź: Wyd. UŁ.

Ogińska-Bulik, N. (2011a). Rola prężności psychicznej w przystosowaniu się kobiet do choroby nowotworowej. *Psychoonkologia*, 1, 26–35.

Ogińska-Bulik, N. (2013). *Pozytywne skutki doświadczeń traumatycznych, czyli kiedy łzy zamieniają się w perły*. Warszawa: Difin.

Ogińska-Bulik, N., Juczyński, Z. (2008). Skala pomiaru prężności – SPP-25. *Nowiny Psychologiczne*, 3, 39–56.

Ogińska-Bulik, N., Juczyński, Z. (2010, wyd. II uzup.). *Osobowość, stres a zdrowie*. Warszawa: Difin.

Ogińska-Bulik, N., Juczyński, Z. (2011). Prężność u dzieci i młodzieży: charakterystyka i pomiar – polska skala SPP-18. *Polskie Forum Psychologiczne*, 16(1), 7–28.

Ostrowski, T.M. (2010). *Sposoby definiowania duchowości w naukach behawioralnych*. [W:] L. Suchocka, R. Sztembis (red.). *Człowiek i dzieło. Księga jubileuszowa dedykowana Księdzu Profesorowi Kazimierzowi Popielskiemu* (269–285). Lublin: Wydawnictwo Katolickiego Uniwersytetu Lubelskiego.

Pargament, K.I. (1997). *The psychology of religion and coping: Theory, research, practice*. New York: The Guilford Press.

Peres, J.F.P., Moreira-Almeida, A., Nasello, A.G., Koenig, H.G. (2007a). Spirituality and resilience in trauma victims. *Journal of Religion and Health*, 46, 343–350.

Peres, J.F.P., Newberg, A.B., Mercante, J.P., Simão, M., Albuquerque, V.E., Peres, M.J., Nasello, A.G. (2007b). Cerebral blood flow changes during retrieval of traumatic memories before and after psychotherapy: aSPECTstudy. *Psychological Medicine*, 37, 1481–91.

Salovey, P., Mayer, J.D. (1989–1990). *Emotional intelligence. Imagination, Cognition, and Personality*, 9, 185–211.

Sęk, H., Cieślak, R. (2004). *Wsparcie społeczne, stres i zdrowie*. Warszawa: Wydawnictwo Naukowe PWN.

Schuster, M.A., Stein, B.D., Jaycox, L., Collins, R.L., Marshall, G.N., Elliott, M.N., Zhou, A.J., Kanouse, D.E., Morrison, J.L., Berry, S.H. (2001). A national survey of stress reactions after the September 11, 2001, terrorist attacks. *The New England Journal of Medicine*, 345, 1507–1512.

Sperry, L. (2001). *Spirituality in clinical practice: Incorporating the spiritual dimension in psychotherapy and counseling*. New York: Brunner-Routledge.

Tugade, M., Fredrickson, B. (2004). Resilient individuals use positive emotions to bounce back from negative emotional experiences. *Journal of Personality and Social Psychology*, 86, 320–333.

Tugade, M., Fredrickson, B., Barrett, L. (2004). Psychological Resilience and Positive Emotional Granularity: Examining the Benefits of Positive Emotions on Coping and Health. *Journal of Personality*, 72, 1161–1190.

Van Dyke, C.J., Elias, M.J. (2007). How forgiveness, purpose, and religiosity are related to the mental health and well-being of youth. A review of literature. *Mental Health Religion Culture*, 10, 395–415.

Vieweg, W.V., Julius, D.A., Fernandez, A., Beatty-Brooks, M., Hettema, J.M., Pandurangi, A.K. (2006). Posttraumatic stress disorder: Clinical features, pathophysiology, and treatment. *American Journal of Medicine*, 119, 383–390.

Werner, E.E. (1996). Vulnerable but invincible: High risk children from birth to adulthood. *European Child, Adolescent Psychiatry*, 5(1), 47–51.

Konrad Banicki
Jagiellonian University
The Institute of Applied Psychology

NATURALISM, NORMATIVISM AND HAVI CAREL'S PHENOMENOLOGICAL APPROACH TO HEALTH AND ILLNESS

> "My body *is* me. This is an essential feature of our embodied existence that is brought out be illness. Illness is an abrupt, violent way of revealing the intimately bodily nature of our being."
>
> Carel, 2008, p. 27

Abstract

The notions of health, disease, and illness as essentially applicable in all medical contexts have been extensively discussed within contemporary philosophy of medicine. Among the variety of perspectives offered there are two which seem to be currently dominating: the naturalistic and the normativist ones. The former approach, as represented by Boorse's biostatistical theory, tends to focus on the notion of disease, which is understood in terms of an impairment of statistically normal biological functioning. The latter one in turn, as developed for instance within the action-theoretical theory of Nordenfelt, denies the possibility of specifying health and illness in purely objective biological terms and provides an openly normative framework which is founded on the notions of human ability and vital goals. These two approaches, though obviously different in many non-negligible aspects, still share one crucial feature: they are formulated from a third-person perspective and use third-person language, accordingly. Having made this point, Carel intended to develop a perspective which would do justice to first-person experiences, especially to those of an ill person. The phenomenological framework offered by her as well as its philosophical sources are briefly scrutinised.

Key words: health, disease, illness, Boorse, Nordenfelt, Carel, biostatistical theory, action-theoretic approach, phenomenology

One of the central purposes of contemporary philosophy of medicine and bioethics is an attempt to delineate and discuss the notions of health, disease and illness (for general introduction see Murphy, 2008). The focus on these particular concepts, importantly, is motivated by their general character and breadth. They can be meaningfully refered, in particular, not only to all these medical contexts in which they explicitly appear but also to those in which they may initially seem to be absent. A particular philosophical position concerning health, diseases and illness; a position which can be implicit, unsystematic, and incoherent, but which still is as a philosophical position, for instance, seems to be inevitable within all discussions of such normatively-ladden concepts as therapy, treatment, recovery, or development. Any serious investigation into the notion of resilience, furthermore, as the one obviously dependend on the concept of normal (healthy) functioning, can also greatly benefit from an explicit discussion of the problematic area of health, disease, and illness.

The attempt to reliably discuss the latter notions, what is more, is not only driven by purely theoretical considerations but also by those of more practical character. The notions in question, in particular, can be easily shown as having a far-reaching consequences for medical practice, a practice for which they determine its specific goal: the removal of disease (illness) and/or the achievement of health. As such they can have a considerable bearing on the whole medical world, not only on the very clinic but also on medical education and politics (including health insurance policy).[1]

One of recent attempts to offer a new approach to the issues of illness and health has been made by the British philosopher Havi Carel in her book titled *Illness. The Cry of the Flesh* (Carel, 2008; cf. Carel, 2011, 2012). The importance of this proposal results not only from its theoretical merits but also from the fact that it is based of the author's own "experience of living with a degenerative and potentially fatal illness: an illness that has no treatment" (Carel, 2008, p. 7).[2] This fact, as one will see in what follows, is especially important within the context of particular approach offered by Carel – the phenomenological one.

The experience of a very serious illness, as Carel (2008, p. 7) herself reports, has pushed her "to reflect abstractly on health and illness" and to ask "what these concepts mean and how best to understand them." What she found out as a result, however, was that the routinely applied medical language is "inappropriate, incomplete and often misleading." One of the direct consequences of this impoverishment of medical conceptual framework, as she believes, is "the inability to speak of important things" and, hence, the need for a new approach

---

[1] For the analysis of health concept's consequences for health care see Nordenfelt (1993).

[2] In 2006 Havi Carel received a diagnosis of lymphangioleiomyomatosis (LAM), a rare cancer-like lung disease. For further information see www.lamtreatmentalliance.org, www.lamaction.org, and www.thelamfoundation.org.

that would enable "us to express the experience of illness" (Carel, 2008, p. 6 and 10, respectively).

While speaking about the "inappropriate, incomplete and often misleading" medical language and concepts Carel refers especially to two particular perspectives that have dominated philosophy of medicine in recent decades: the naturalistic and normativist ones. *The naturalistic approach* to disease and health, to begin with, can be called an orthodox or mainstream one within the contemporary medical world. The naturalism of this approach refers to the fact that it conceives the human being as, entirely or at least primarily, "a complicated biological organism with a vast number of interacting parts" (Nordenfelt, 1986, p. 281). Human diseases, accordingly, are perceived as fully belonging to the natural world and, hence, as exhaustively describable and explainable in naturalistic terms, such as those of physics, biology, and chemistry.

Even thought medical naturalism is an umbrella term that covers a relatively broad spectrum of perspectives, it is *the biostatistical theory* developed by Christopher Boorse (1975, 1977, 1997; cf. Cooper, 2002) that seems to be dominating, both as a source of positive inspiration and as an aim of naturalism's critics. A *disease*, according to this proposal, can be identified with "a type of internal state which is either an impairment of normal functional ability, i.e. a reduction of one or more functional abilities below typical efficiency, or a limitation on functional ability caused by environmental agents." *Health*, in turn, is nothing more than "the absence of disease" (Boorse, 1977, p. 567). The theoretical cornerstone of this definition is the concept of *functional ability*, which, in turn, is based on the notions of survival and reproduction. A normal function of a bodily organ or system, more particularly, is its contribution to the individual's survival and reproduction, which is statistically typical of a respective *reference class*, i.e., a class of organisms of the same species, sex, and age as the one in question.

A crucial feature of Boorse's theory, as well as the one that makes it an instance of an objectivist approach (cf. Murphy, 2008), is that it conceives the notions of disease and health as essentially "value-free and descriptive in the same sense as the concepts of atom, metal and rain are value-free and descriptive" (Nordenfelt, 2007, p. 5). The diagnosis of an organism as diseased, accordingly, is a matter of discovering some biochemical facts. It can be objectively made by standard medical and scientific procedures, without the necessity of referring to any normative issues.

The fact that Boorse's approach is currently dominant is not accidental. The biostatistical theory is certainly sophisticated, well-organised and quantitative. Also, as even its critics admit, it has many considerable advantages. Nordenfelt (2007, p. 6), for example, points to the fact that its reliance on the concepts of survival and reproduction makes it not only well-fitted into the evolutionary framework but also easily applicable to non-humans including animals from apes to "worms and amoebas" and plants "from orchids to mosses." Even despite of these indisputable advantages, however, the biostatistical perspective, or naturalistic approach to the phenomena of disease and health in general, has been subjected to substantial criticism (see especially Nordenfelt, 1995). It has been argued, for instance, that it underestimates the environmental and inter-individual variations of human functioning as well as the extent to which one subnormal function can be compensated by another supernormal one.

The most important doubt, however, concerns Boorse's consistency in providing a value-free account. Or, more significantly, it is the very possibility of addressing the issues of health and disease without presuming any normative viewpoint that is put into question. The whole family of the approaches that deny such a possibility can be conveniently subsumed under the heading of normativism.

The most general tenet, common to all *normativist approaches*, is that the notions of health and disease are essentially value-laden. These notions, more particularly, are believed to be inevitably entangled with normative presumptions concerning human behaviour and/or well-being. To say that somebody suffers from a disease, in consequence, is something more than to objectively diagnose this person's bodily functions. Contrary to the views of the naturalists, it is also non-accidentally to make a normative statement concerning the undesirability of these functions' current state as well as its behavioural and experiential consequences.

Normativism, importantly, conceives the human as "fundamentally a social agent, a complete human being acting in society" (Nordenfelt, 1986, p. 281). As soon as one takes such a perspective, significantly, the notions of biochemical and physical kind turn out to be principally insufficient to describe and account for a human being, including an ill human being. These are the value-laden concepts derived from social sciences and the humanities, instead, that need to be applied.

One of the most often debated version of normativism has been proposed by Lennart Nordenfelt (1995, cf. 1986, 1993, 2007) as so called *holistic* or *action-theoretical approach*. Within a framework of theory of action and essentially social view of human being, in particular, *health* has been defined as "a person's ability, in standard circumstances, to reach his vital goals" (Nordenfelt, 1995, p. 145). A *disease*, in turn, has been conceived as physical or mental process "which is such that it tends to reduce its bearer's health" (Nordenfelt, 1993, p. 280).

The notion which is crucial to the above-given definitions is the one of *vital goals* as "those states of affairs the realization of which are necessary and jointly sufficient" (Nordenfelt, 1995, p. 145) for the *minimal welfare* of a person in question. Its importance lies in the fact that it is the seat of the health and disease notion's normativity. The exact character of minimal welfare, in particular, is left undetermined. The question concerning the latter "is not a question of science" (Nordenfelt, 1995, p. 78). It has to "be decided upon, and cannot simply be the result of empirical investigation" (Nordenfelt, 1995, p. xvi). This necessity of referring to so called *primary evaluation* (Nordenfelt, 1995, p. 78, italics added) while determining the particular content of the health concept is a feature that most directly reflects the essentially normative character of the latter.[3]

If one wanted to set the biostatistical and action-theoretical approaches together, one would obviously found a lot of non-trivial differences (Nordenfelt, 1986, 1993, 2007). The perspective offered by Boorse, to begin with, is founded on the notion of disease (the concept of health is defined in negative terms) and specified in terms which are derived from biology and statistics. The health-related goals of an organism, accordingly, are the ones of reproduction and survival. Both health and disease, furthermore, are believed to be purely objective matters to be determined by scientific methods. Nordenfelt's approach, in turn, is built on the concept of health (the one of disease is derivative) and applies conceptual framework which is proper to social sciences including the terms such as those of goal or welfare. Human vital goals, importantly, are understood as significantly broader than pure survival, which they include as "a necessary condition for the accomplishment of all other goals" (Nordenfelt, 2007, p. 9). The phenomena of health and disease as viewed from this perspective, finally, are explicitly and consequently depicted as value-laden.

All these differences can be hardly overemphasised. Still, however, there is an important formal feature that these both approaches share and that has become the origin of Carel's criticism directed at them. The characteristic in question is a *third-person perspective and language* employed by these two proposals. The *first-person perspective*, including the first-person experience of an ill person, accordingly, seems to be non-accidentally and seriously neglected.

It is exactly due to this neglect that the *Illness*' author, even though having admitted that the accounts summarized above "both have merits and have spawned a large literature," insists that there is "a different set of issues pertaining to illness that is not captured by either approach (Carel, 2008, p. 12). What is principally excluded by them, more particularly, is "the experience of being ill: illness as it is lived by the ill person." Illness, as Carel argues, is not only a disease, i.e. an abnormal bodily state or process. It is also, or even primarily, a first-person physical, psychological and social experience including the experience of the life changes that disease may entail. Both naturalism and normativism, with all the non-trivial differences between these two models, are both substantially unable to address these kind of issues: "the world of the ill person," in Carel's (2008, p. 12) own words, "is not heard."

It is with this critical diagnosis of currently dominating approaches to health and disease and their ability of doing justice to "the world of the ill person" in

---

[3] Another case, in which this normativeness is visible, is the fact that the notion of standard circumstances used is the definition of health is different from the one of statistically normal environment (proper to Boorse's approach). Standard circumstances, in particular, "are related to a cultural norm" (Nordenfelt, 2007, p. 7).

mind that Carel attempted at finding a language and conceptual framework that would be more appropriate to let the patient speak for him/herself. The place in which she found what she was looking for was *philosophical phenomenology*.

Having said this, there are at least two remarks that have to be necessarily made. Phenomenology, at first, is a very complex and internally heterogeneous philosophical movement, which used to to be associated with such diverse figures as Franz Brentano (cf. his idea of descriptive psychology), Edmund Husserl, or Martin Heidegger. Even Husserl, i.e. the very founder of the movement, cannot be simply connected with one particular idea of phenomenology, because his approach had substantially evolved. This considerable heterogeneity should be always kept in mind in the context of Carel's presentation, which usually does not dwell much on technicalities.[4] The second remark that could be made concerns the closer context of Carel's project. The idea of applying phenomenology to the experience of illness and health, in particular, is shared by her with some other interesting thinkers such as Richard Zaner (1981, 2005), S. Kay Toombs (1987, 1993), or Fredrik Svenaeus (2000, 2001).

The phenomenological idea that has been of crucial appeal to Carel can be easily derived from the very name of the current: "the phenomenology." Phenomenology as understood etymologically, in particular, is nothing less that the science (gr. *logos*) of what is in the most general sense experienced, i.e. of the *phenomena*. What is especially significant is the fact that phenomenology has explicitly first-person and descriptive character. It is "a descriptive philosophical method" (Carel, 2011, p. 34) that focuses on direct individual experiences without any ambitions to go beyond them. Not only are all possible philosophical and scientific explanations of what (and how) is experienced put into bracket, but also the very reality of experienced things is put aside. The phenomenologist, accordingly, is interested in "things (*phenomena*) *as they appear to us*," not in the things themselves (Carel, 2008, p. 10).

When applied to illness, it would mean that it is the lived experience of a suffering person, his/her acts of consciousness, experiences, and perceptions, rather then scientifically, third-personally and objectively specified biochemical fact of disease, that will be put to the fore. In the cases of serious and/or chronic illnesses, what is more, *the phenomenology of illness* will focus on these experiences as more holistically and globally structured, i.e. on the "illness as a way of living, experiencing the world and interacting with other people" (Carel, 2008, p. 8).

---

[4] Understandably, it is mostly the case of the book (Carel, 2008), which is aimed at general audience, rather than the texts written mostly for scholars (Carel, 2011, 2012). In her paper from 2011, for instance, Carel admits that within phenomenology "there are different views and emphases" and that phenomenology itself is "normally described as a transcendental mode of inquire" (p. 34 and 35, respectively). The latter remark is especially important, because the transcendental thread, crucial as it was for Husserl, is not usually regarded important by the author of *Illness* (cf. "For the purposes of describing the experience of illness, it is enough to consider the general features of illness without insisting on the transcendental nature of its features," Carel, 2011, p. 35).

Phenomenology as it is conceived by Carel (2008, p. 71) is first of all "a view that enables a complete description of the ways in which the life and world of the ill person changes." As such, importantly, it is not intended to "displace" the thirdperson perspectives such as naturalism and normativism. It is meant, rather, to "*augment*" them or, in the words of Svenaeus (2001, p. 87), to "enrich our understanding of health in adding to the disease-level analysis a level of analysis that addresses the question how the physiological states are lived as meaningful in an environment."

Within the whole bunch of phenomenological approaches it was the French philosopher Maurice Merleau-Ponty that turned out to be the most helpful for the Carel's attempt. The reason for which she found this philosopher "particularly compelling in relation to illness" (Carel, 2008, p. 20) was his view of human lived experience and existence as substantially *embodied* and founded on *perception*. The body and perception, as seen by Merleau-Ponty in particular, are "the seat of personhood, or subjectivity" (Carel, 2008, p. 20), the "*sine qua non* of human existence" (Carel, 2011, p. 37). Any change affecting the body and/or perception can and, in fact, must influence the very subjectivity itself. The human being, what is more, is always *enworlded*, i.e. substantially related to the meaningful world he/she perceives and in which he/she acts: "a perceiving and experiencing organism, intimately inhabiting and immediately responding to her environment" (Carel, 2008, p. 20).

This view of human subjectivity and personhood has many non-negligible consequences. The most general of them concerns epistemological issues. It turns out, in particular, that any theoretical attempt aiming at the understanding of the human has to be founded on thick enough account of body and perception as the foundations of the self or, in slightly more concise terms, on the idea of the human "both as having a body and as having a world" (Carel, 2008, p. 13). Any perspective that does not include these dimensions will be simply "a deficient account."

The approach offered by Merleau-Ponty, significantly, is through and through *anti-dualistic* and, in a sense, *anti-intellectual*. As such it can be directly contrasted with the views of Descartes who famously conceived the human as essentially a mind or a soul (Latin *res cogitas*, or thinking substance) which is only contingently connected with a body (Latin *res extensa*, or extended substance). Descartes' dualism, as one may remember, is one of the two founding principles of contemporary biomedical, or naturalistic, medical paradigm (see Engel, 1977; the second presumption is reductionism). Phenomenological approach, accordingly, will remain in essential tension with the latter. Anti-dualism of Merleau-Ponty, when stated in more positive terms, can be identified as a *holistic* position which emphasises "the inseparability of mind and body, of thinking and perceiving" (Carel, 2008, p. 21). Consciousness and mental activity, in short, even in their most subtle and abstract forms, are always both embodied and mediated by perception.

The rejection of dualism, interestingly, affects not only the view of the mind (soul) but also that of the body. The Cartesian body was significantly passive: a material being susceptible to the commands of active and intentional mind.[5] By itself it was nothing more than a mechanism "that only comes to life when infused with a soul" (Carel, 2008, p. 21). Within Merleau-Ponty's perspective, to compare with, the body is as 'ensouled' as the soul is embodied. The body, in particular, is not only active in a general sense of the term, but also "an intelligent, planning, and goal-oriented entity" (Carel, 2008, p. 38), an entity that is permanently engaged in meaningful relationships with the world it inhabits. This body, as a matter of fact, can be quite literally assigned the property of intentionality.

The body as seen by Merleau-Ponty, what is more, is unique in that aspect that it "can be experienced both from a third-person point of view... and from a first-person point of view" (Carel, 2008, p. 23). When the former perspective is taken, the body is simply a physical or material object: the *biological body* (ger. *der Körper*, franc. *le corps objectif*) that can be subjected to standard scientific procedures including weighing, measuring, and inspection. It can be described and accounted for, accordingly, in objective terms derived from natural sciences including biologically understood medicine. What is crucial, however, is the fact that it is always something more than this. When conceived from a subjective perspective, namely, the body becomes "the first-person experience of the biological body... the body as lived by the person" (Carel, 2008, p. 26).

The notion of the *lived body* (ger. *Der Leib*, franc. *le corps propre*) is of central importance here, because it represents the whole potential of phenomenological approach to illness. A healthy biological body, to begin with, is usually transparent: it is either not experienced at all or remains in the experiential background. As long as everything goes smoothly, this body is taken for granted in the very same sense in which an efficient instrument is taken for granted while utilizing it. The biological body and the body as lived "are aligned, in harmony." (Carel, 2011, p. 39). When something adverse and/or surprising happens to the biological body, however, this harmony becomes disrupted. When a body part rejects to cooperate, for instance, our awareness is "drawn to the malfunctioning body part and suddenly it [this body part, KB] becomes the focus of our attention, rather than the invisible background for our activities... It ceases to be an invisible background enabling some projects and becomes a stubborn saboteur instead" (Carel, 2008, p. 26).

A crucial point to make is that illness is one of the most obvious examples of this kind of collision. Its crucial aspect is the fact that an ill person begins to feel

---

[5] An exact way in which this relationship between two substantially different substances can be at all possible was obviously very mysterious. The vicissitudes of so called body-mind problem is the best evidence for that.

estranged from his/her own body[6] and is, in a sense, removed "from the normal flux of life" (Carel, 2012, p. 104).[7] The illness, in general, can be potentially full of very tremendous and far-reaching consequences to the person him/herself. As such, accordingly, it turns out to be nothing less than "a painful and violent way of revealing the intimately bodily nature of our being" (Carel, 2011, p. 40).

Necessarily concise remarks made above can be a good illustration of the way in which Merleau-Ponty's idea of the lived body as something distinct from the biological one provides a conceptual tool, by which we can express an insight that illness in not only, or even not primarily, an isolated fact concerning human physiology, but a phenomenon that substantially affects the embodied person as a whole, including his/her relationships to the environment. Illness, as a result, turns out to be a situation in which "one's entire way of being in the world is altered" (Carel, 2008, p. 73). And it is exactly the task of doing justice to the experience of this tremendous change that cannot be done by any third-person approach and that is the point at which phenomenology can reveal all its merits and potential. The shift in one's existence imposed by illness, as Carel (2008, p. 29) emphasises, "is not local but global, not external but strikes at the heart of subjectivity." This truth applies especially to severe and/or chronic diseases (as well as to disability). The conditions of this kind, accordingly, are hardly addressable by any approach that does not include a comprehensive and consistent account of the embodied self. It is only "through embodied phenomenology," in brief, that "the tremendous impact of illness becomes visible" (Carel, 2011, p. 41).

The experience of illness, obviously, can take a great number of different shapes. Still, however, it seems to be possible to identify some features which are common to all, or at least to the majority of them. Before Carel, an attempt at identifying these features has been made by Toombs (1993, p. 90) who developed a list of *the essential characteristics of the experience of illness* including "a loss of wholeness, a loss of certainty, a loss of control, a loss of freedom to act, and a loss of the familiar world." This list has been supplemented by the author of *Illness* with "three additional themes" (Carel, 2012, p. 103): (1) the changes in the way space and time is experienced, (2) lost abilities, and (3) adaptability. The distinctions between the characteristics and themes proper to illness, importantly, should not be interpreted as implying that this experience can be "compartmentalized into discrete areas" (Carel, 2012, p. 102). These features, quite oppositely, are only dimensions of ultimately unitary and global phenomenon. In serious and/or chronic conditions, even more, they can be conceived as aspects of an illness that has become "a complete form of life" (Carel, 2012, p. 97).

---

[6] Cf. Svenaeus' (2000, 2001) application of the notion of „Unheimlichkeit" as a state in which one is not at home in one's own lived body.

[7] This removal, as Carel (2012, p. 104) notices, is not only due to the confinements of bodily abilities connected with a disease, but also "because of social and psychological barriers to participation, for example, embarrassment or anxiety."

(1) The modification concerning *the experience of time and space*, to begin with, can be understood as these two dimensions of the experienced physical world becoming "less welcoming, full of obstacles, difficult" (Carel, 2012, p. 103). When one is ill, distances which used to be short increase. Tasks which used to take a short time require a considerably longer one. These changes are especially vivid in the cases of disability, such as those requiring one to use a wheelchair. Even common headache or sore feet, however, can lead a person to the experience of time and distance to be walked as both painfully long.

Toombs (1993, p. 97) writes that illness "truncates experiencing" in its spatio-temporal dimension. The "unavoidable preoccupation with pain, sickness, or incapacity, grounds one in the present moment" and makes the future "suddenly disabled, rendered impotent and inaccessible." The space, similarly, becomes considerably confined ("to the bed, to the house, to the hospital") and restrictive ("a location may be 'too far' from the bed or chair, a step 'too high' to climb, a room 'too crowded' to navigate"). Diagnosis, especially a diagnosis of an illness with uncertain prognosis, as Carel adds, may confront one with limited time given to a fragile and mortal human being. As such, in turn, it may lead to the reconsideration of one's values and commitments and give "an opportunity to consider how one has lived and how one would like to live" (Carel, 2012, p. 104).

(2) The second of the themes explored by Carel are *lost abilities*. A healthy body is, first of all, an able body, a body that remains transparent and taken for granted just because it is able to be engaged in the tasks that capture whole attention. An ill body, on the other hands, "thwarts plans, impedes choices, renders actions impossible" (Toombs, 1993, p. 90). The idea of embodied existence, as one may remember, posits that all goal-directed activity, including one directed at even the most abstract goals, is necessarily mediated by bodily action, including perception. Any weakness of the body or the restriction of physical and perceptual potential, respectively, is inevitably connected with the confinement of one's ability to "assert oneself, perform actions and carry out activities that promote one's goals" (Carel, 2008, p. 73). As such, it does transform the very heart of the self, the agent's subjectivity and global existence.

(3) The illness as lived, importantly, although it may seem to be constituted by negative dimensions only (cf. the Toombs' list of losses mentioned above), can also involve more positive aspects among which there are *creative responses* to all that have been lost. The process of *adaptability*, in general, is directed at the discovery of new ways to achieve old goals and, as such, can be very broad and global. In many cases, as a matter of fact, it can be understood as aiming at the discovery (or invention?) of a completely new way of being, a way in which a person can be happy and lead a worthwhile life despite the fact that he/she is seriously ill. Creative reactions to illness, importantly, apart from their intrinsic and direct value, can also lead to some further positive outcomes such as a sense of achievement while coping with obstacles, the feeling of joy about the present,

serene attitude towards one's adverse circumstances, or a deeper insight into the human condition with all its fragility and accidentality. These kind of outcomes are often subsumed under the heading of "health within illness" (Lindsey, 1996).

The very possibility of *health within illness* revealed by phenomenological analyses, as Carel argues, entails the necessity of making a considerable conceptual shift. Health and illness, to begin with, can no longer be conceived as mutually exclusive and opposite to each other. They should be rather conceived in terms of "a continuum or a blend of the two, allowing for health within illness in people who seem objectively ill" (Carel, 2008, p. 78). A business-as-usual assessment focused on objectively measured deficits, what is more, should be supplemented by more first-person approach which would let the patients, who often report positive aspects even while suffering very serious diseases, to speak. The most general insight gained by the application of phenomenological viewpoint is that "illness is part and parcel of life, and on a continuum with health" (Carel, 2008, p. 80). The traditional model of medical thinking and healthcare practice built around the notions of disease and cure, as a result, should be at least complemented by more positive one emphasising health and well-being promotion as well as healing.

The necessary conceptual shift summarized above, as Carel argues, can and should be followed by particular *applications* referring not only to medical training and practice, but also to the study of therapeutic outcomes, or methodological issues (Carel, 2011).

Medical training, for instance, is currently founded on the biomedical model with all its reductionism and mechanism. As such it has certainly proved to be very efficient in many areas. Still, however, it is completely impotent as far as the global and subjective experience of illness is concerned, which makes the illness as lived "unacknowledged within clinical medicine" (Carel, 2012, p. 98). Phenomenological perspective, on the other hand, if it was included into medical training could help such acknowledgement happen. It could, for example, be applied as a medium through which the clinicians could become aware of the common features of illness, such as those enumerated by Toombs and Carel. New insights and sensibilities, accordingly, could be developed and the general ability to empathise increased.

The biomedical conceptual model, significantly, not only hinders health care professionals in their attempts to understand patients, but also has a very serious impact on the latter. In fact, it could be hard to overemphasise "the extent to which patients' own understanding of their illness is influenced by medical attitudes and their encounters with the health care system" (Carel, 2012, p. 98). Medical staff is the primary source from which patients obtain the information about their maladies. While receiving these information, importantly, patients are not only provided with facts concerning their condition but also with a particular discourse, in which they learn, are taught, to think about themselves. This biomedical discourse, importantly, can seriously confine the ability of addressing the subjective and existential dimension of an illness and, as such, "may lead to a sense of alienation and a lack of a first-person voice in patients' discourse about their illness" (Carel, 2012, p. 98).

A remedy for this situation, according to Carel (2012, p. 99), can be provided by the phenomenological perspective with its avowedly descriptive, i.e. non-prescriptive and non-explanatory, and first-person approach which makes it "uniquely suited to the exploration of the experience of illness" with all its far-reaching consequences to the very subjectivity of a patient and his/her way of being. The author of *Illness*, as a matter of fact, has recently initiated the development of "a *phenomenological toolkit* that can be offered to patients as a workshop" (Carel, 2012, p. 97, italics added). This toolkit, more specifically, would provide patients with phenomenological language and viewpoint helping them to describe and order their experience of illness.[8] A new perspective on illness gained by the application of this toolkit, furthermore, could be subsequently presented to health care professionals and "help construct a shared meaning of illness" (Carel, 2011, p. 42).

The development of a phenomenological toolkit, apart from its most straightforward character and merits, can be understood as a point at which Carel comes back to the most direct reality of illness. A considerable part of her work has been devoted to relatively distanced and abstracted investigations into the themes of illness and health. It is in this part that she introduced the phenomenological viewpoint and argued for its importance for the medical discourse and practice currently dominated by third-person approaches of naturalism and normativism. Still, however, the ultimate goal of her work was connected with real people, whose illnesses she hoped to make "a little less scary, less anonymous" (Carel, 2008, p. 18).

While concluding her book Havi Carel (2008, p. 134) wrote: "Illness can be a journey. Like some journeys, you do not always know where it will take you. This particular journey moved from personal experiences of illness to a philosophical exploration of their meaning." One of the things that she wanted to convey was that her reflections on illness had been neither exclusively philosophical and, hence, mostly third-personal and objective, nor solely personal and subjective. Phenomenology as depicted by her, in other words, is "a theory that has become a lived experience and is then rethought in light of experience" (Carel, 2008, p. 117). This "sometimes difficult" (Carel, 2008, p. 13) attempt at remaining simultaneously committed to both first- and third-person approaches is certainly one of the features that makes her account that precious.

An important point to be made is that by the very same token the brief presentation of the phenomenological approach offered in this chapter, a presentation

---

[8] The workshop, interestingly, is also intended to include "nonlinguistic means for self-description and self-reflection" (Carel, 2012, p. 109) such as collage or a song.

that has been made in an objective and third-person manner, is inevitably one-sided and limited. This kind of fundamental confinement can be remedied only within more personal perspective such as that proper to experience or genuine interpersonal dialogue.

References

Boorse, C. (1975). On the distinction between health and illness. *Philosophy and Public Affairs*, 5, 49–68.
Boorse, C. (1977). Health as a theoretical concept. *Philosophy of Science*, 44, 542–573.
Boorse, C. (1997). *A rebuttal on health*. [In:] J.M. Humber, R.F. Almeder (Eds.). *What is disease?* (pp. 3–143). Totowa, New York: Humana Press.
Carel, H. (2008). *Illness. The cry of the flesh*. Durham: Acumen Publishing.
Carel, H. (2011). Phenomenology and its application in medicine. *Theoretical Medicine and Bioethics*, 32, 33–46.
Carel, H. (2012). Phenomenology as a resource for patients. *Journal of Medicine and Philosophy*, 37, 96–113.
Cooper, R. (2002). Disease. *Studies in History and Philosophy of Biological and Biomedical Sciences*, 33, 263–282.
Engel, G.L. (1977). The need for a new medical model: a challenge for biomedicine. *Science*, 196, 129–136.
Lindsey, E. (1996). Health within illness: experiences of chronically ill/disabled people. *Journal of Advanced Nursing*, 24, 465–472.
Murphy, D. (2008). *Concepts of disease and health*. [In:] E.N. Zalta (Ed.). *The Stanford Encyclopedia of Philosophy* (*Summer 2009 Edition*) (http://plato.stanford.edu/archives/sum2009/entries/health-disease).
Nordenfelt, L. (1986). Health and disease: two philosophical perspectives. *Journal of Epidemiology and Community Health*, 41, 281–284.
Nordenfelt, L. (1993). Concepts of health and their consequences for health care. *Theoretical Medicine*, 14, 277–285.
Nordenfelt, L. (1995). *On the nature of health. An action-theoretic approach*. Dordrecht: Kluwer Academic Publishers.
Nordenfelt, L. (2007). The concepts of health and illness revisited. *Medicine, Health Care and Philosophy*, 10, 5–10.
Svenaeus, F. (2000). *The hermeneutics of medicine and the phenomenology of health*. Dordrecht: Kluwer Academic Publishers.
Svenaeus, F. (2001). *The phenomenology of health and illness*. [In:] S.K. Toombs (Eds.). *Handbook of phenomenology and medicine* (87–108). Dordrecht: Kluwer Academic Publishers.
Toombs, S.K. (1987). The meaning of illness: a phenomenological approach to the patient-physician relationship. *The Journal of Medicine and Philosophy*, 12, 219–240.
Toombs, S.K. (1993). *The meaning of illness. A phenomenological account of the different perspectives of physician and patient*. Dordrecht: Kluwer Academic Publishers.
Zaner, R.M. (1981). *The context of self: a phenomenological inquiry using medicine as a clue*. Athens, OH: Ohio University Press.
Zaner, R.M. (2005). A work in progress. *Theoretical Medicine*, 26, 89–104.

Krzysztof Gerc
Jagiellonian University
The Institute of Applied Psychology

TESTING THE SENSE OF IDENTITY IN PEOPLE WITH HIGHLY FUNCTIONING AUTISM AS THEORY-METHODOLOGICAL PROBLEM

Abstract

This article refers to the paradigm of cognitive and developmental psychology and triadic concept of identity of L. Witkowski. It presents basic problems referring to, among other things, the psychological characterizing of sense of identity in people with highly functioning autism.
Referring to contemporary, existing in literature theoretic solutions and empiric analysis of operating of people with highly functioning autism, in this article there will be discussed briefly three suggested by Witkowski scopes of identity – that is competence, concept and condition. The last part of the article will be dedicated to the example case of adolescent with highly functioning autism and pointing at diagnostic and interpretation difficulties which appeared while using commonly used psychological tools in psychological guidance.

Key words: high-functioning autism, sense of identity

Introduction

The end of the 20th century has brought remarkable advances in the research and theory concerning the issues of autism. Researchers representing various theoretical frameworks contributed to a more comprehensive approach to the disorder, which allowed to adequately describe the autism spectrum disorders, as well as to pick up the complex issue of identity research in people with high-functioning autism.

The descriptions of the autism spectrum disorders contained in two international classifications – ICD-10 and DSM-IV-TR – are currently convergent. However, the diagnostic criteria of the Asperger syndrome in the aforementioned classifications differ markedly in some respects from criteria put forward by individual researchers, particularly with respect to the development of speech and language. C. Gillberg (2005) and P. Szatmari (2000) point to non-typical characteristics of speech and language in children with the Asperger syndrome, or features of the so-called eccentric speech, while the ICD-10 and DSM-IV-TR criteria include no such characteristics.

In the category of autistic disorders, the DSM-IV distinguishes five of them: Autistic Disorder, Rett's Disorder, Childhood Disintegrative Disorder, Asperger's Disorder and Pervasive Developmental Disorder Not Otherwise Specified.

In the work in progress, scheduled for publication in May 2013, the latest version of the Diagnostic-Statistic Handbook of Psychological Disorders (DSM-V), important changes are proposed with respect to the classification of autism and the Asperger syndrome. It is intended to include autistic disorders, defined as Autism Spectrum Disorders (ASDs), in the group of neurodevelopmental disorders already present in the classification. The category will contain disorders formerly referred to as the autistic disorder, Asperger's disorder, childhood disintegrative disorder, and the pervasive developmental disorder not otherwise specified Considering the above propositions, the APA suggests the removal of Asperger disorder from the DSM-V classification, justifying the suggestion, among others, with empirical analyses that indicate that the application of the diagnostic criteria of the Asperger disorder in clinical practice often was not reliable. The APA recommends the changes referring to conclusions reached by renowned researchers of the problem, such as Mayes et al., 2001; Miller, Ozonoff, 2000; Leekam, Libby, Wing, Gould, Gillberg, 2000 (after: Attwood, 2006).

It seems that the removal of Asperger syndrome from the classification and the inclusion of the Autism Spectrum Disorders category may have positive as well as negative implications. The absence of a separate diagnostic unit will perhaps contribute to the social reception of the Asperger syndrome as a distinctness caused by slightly higher intensity of certain autistic features than in the general population. On the other hand, the inclusion of people with the Asperger syndrome in the broad category of autistic people may cause additional stigmatization and auto-stigmatization, as the social image of this group will become more ambiguous, and its social reception will be influenced by the stereotype of a person with the Kanner variety of autism, characterized by a lowered intelligence quotient and significant problems with verbal communication.

As noted by J. Crocker and D.M. Quinn, "to be 'stigmatized' is to have social identity (or to belong to a particular social category) that questions the completeness of humanity: the stigmatized has a lesser value in the eyes of other people, is somebody crippled, imperfect" (Crocker, Quinn, 2008, p. 149).

The research of the problems of identity in people with the Asperger syndrome and high-functioning autism, performed based on the concept of *resilience* (Lathar, 2006; Lathar, Zelazzo, 2003; Craig et al., 2003; Sameroff, Rosenblum, 2006; Kumpfer, Summerhays, 2006), has one more essential aspect.

Some studies show the problem of anguish, intensified in people included in this group in the adolescence, manifesting itself as an increase in the number of co-existing depressive disorders, anxiety disorders, and suicidal tendencies. Researchers usually connect them to the experience of peer violence and social rejection (Shtayermman, 2007), but there also appear ideas related to the influence of the stigma (handicap) on the functioning of adolescents with the Asperger syndrome and high-functioning autism (Shtayermman, 2009).

In this approach, resilience (Yates et al., 2003) is interpreted as a dynamic development process by which people acquire the ability to use effectively the internal and external resources to good adaptation, despite the previous experience or the present specific difficulties (e.g. barriers stemming from disability). Therefore, the resilience is understood as a positive or protective process that can reduce the maladjustment of the individual who experience the adversities in life (Greenberg, 2006).

Cognitive theories of autism and the issues of identity

In the paper "Does the autistic child have a 'theory of mind'?" S. Baron-Cohen, U. Frith, and A.M. Leslie presented an outline of the theory of mind (ToM), as well as concepts of its deficits in autism. They adopted the assumptions of a metapresentational theory of pretense by A.M. Leslie that relates the idea of the development of II level representation to the mechanism of the "theory of mind" proposed by D. Premack and G. Woodruff in 1978. In the majority of people there develops a representation of reality which influences all activities of the individual, as well as an awareness that interpretation of certain facts and events is different in different people. According to D. Premack and G. Woodruff, the appearance of this awareness constitute an important step in the social development, and indirectly in the forming of identity (Baron-Cohen et al., 1985). I level representations, characterized by a direct semantic relation to the outside world, concern the physical properties of individual objects and events, while II level representations (metarepresentations), allowing one to create abstract associations, relate, among others, to cognitive and emotional processes in oneself and others (Leslie, 1987; Talarowska et al., 2010). D. Premack and G. Woodruff in turn introduced the notion of the "theory of mind" as a definition of a cognitive mechanism that allows one to infer about mental states in other people (Pisula, 2000).

A.M. Leslie refers to a logical analysis of the properties of assertions introduced with mental state verbs, such as "believe," "expect," or "want," conducted by W.V. Quine. Assertions introduced with these verbs show the following characteristics:

(1) referential opacity – two terms are referentially opaque to each other if they cannot be applied interchangeably without changing the truth-value of the assertion;

(2) nonentailment of truth or falsehood;

(3) nonentailment of existence (or nonexistence).

According to A.M. Leslie's pretense theory, the metarepresentational context separates a copy of a I level representation from its typical transformations of the type input data-output data. An object/situation therefore functions at two levels: a literal level I of representation, where it retains its direct reference to reality, as well as implied judgments about truth and existence, and on level II of representations, deprived of these features (Leslie, 1987; 1992).

Interpreted along these lines, an ability to create meta-representations during childhood is a basis for the cognitive and social development which is a condition of identity forming. Deficits shown in these areas by people with autism have inspired S. Baron-Cohen, U. Frith, and A.M. Leslie to use A.M. Leslie's theory of metarepresentational theory of pretense to explain the axial symptoms of autism. S. Baron-Cohen, U. Frith and A.M. Leslie showed in the research that most probably at the source of problems with cognitive and social situational functioning of people with autism lie deficits in one of basic metarepresentational capability referred to as the "theory of mind" (Baron-Cohen, Frith and Leslie, 1987; Leslie, 1992).

S. Baron-Cohen expanded this concept into a theory based on the assumption that a mind-reading system (MRS) has developed to enable the attribution of mental states to subjects of interaction. It is therefore a "social brain," or "naive psychology," allowing one to formulate explanations of people's behavior as well as predictions of their actions, and as such indispensable for an involvement in social situations. This system in its most advanced form comprises four modular components: ID, EDD, SAM and TOMM; Baron-Cohen acknowledges that ID and TOMM had been described before by, respectively, D. Premack and A.M. Leslie, while he considers the EDD and SAM components as an original part of his theory (Baron-Cohen, *ibid.*; Baron-Cohen, Hadwin, Howlin, 2010; Pisula, 2000). Table 1 shows a general characteristics of individual components of the mind-reading system.

Table 1. Mind Reading System

MRS component	Characteristics
ID (Intentionality Detector)	A primitive perceptional mechanism, interpreting stimuli in terms of target (object of an action) or wish (movement to or from the stimulus) connected with it.
EDD (Eye Direction Detector)	This component has two functions: – detection of eyes or stimuli similar to them; – (in higher primates) representation of eye behavior (e.g. maintaining eye contact).
SAM (Shared Attention Mechanism)	Its role is to determine whether the attention of the subject and another organism in its proximity is focused on the same object, event, etc. This question, an adaptively significant one, cannot be solved by using the ID or EDD components, since they only create binary (dyadic) representations. SAM is therefore necessary for behavior that requires sharing attention. It also performs two other functions: it links the ID and EDD components, and activates the TOMM.
TOMM (Theory of Mind Mechanism)	A system that constitutes the basis of attributing meanings to actions by applying terms denoting mental states, as well as for predicting them. Its two main functions are: (1) representing an array of mental states, including epistemic attitudes, and (2) integrating the knowledge about mental states into a consistent, useful and applicable „theory."

Source: own work, after Baron-Cohen, 1985; Pisula, 2000.

An important issue within the Mind-Reading System theory are the relations among the four components of the system. According to S. Baron-Cohen, a significant difference between the first three mechanisms and the TOMM lies in the fact that the ID, EDD and SAM represent a small group of mental states that only possess two characteristics of Intentionality: *aboutness* (the mental states refer to matters other than themselves) and *aspectuality* (the states refer to specific aspects of their objects). TOMM in turn represents concepts of attitudes, expressed, among others, by such mental state verbs as *pretend, know*, or *believe*. Mental states represented by the TOMM therefore feature a third property of Intentionality – *a possibility of misrepresentation* – that is, a phenomenon earlier referred to by Leslie as the *referential opacity*. S. Baron-Cohen also claims that the TOMM is activated by data (in a tertiary representation) received by means of the SAM component.

S. Baron-Cohen assumed that from among people with autism there can be distinguished two subgroups, characterized by a difference in deficits in the SAM and TOMM areas, which might explain the difference in the time of appearance of early autism signs (before or after the 18th month of life):

Subgroup A: both the SAM and the TOMM are significantly restricted, what is explained by the author in terms of a "domino effect," consisting of the necessity of the development of the SAM component for the TOMM component to function. People in this group show autistic features before the 18th month of life.

Subgroup B: the SAM component is present, while the TOMM is significantly restricted. People in this group develop normally until the 18th month of life, and then start to show autistic features (Baron-Cohen, 1985, 2010; Pisula, 2000).

To sum up, the concept of a mind theory deficit in the autistic spectrum disorders assumes that an underdeveloped mind theory is responsible for the axial symptoms of autism. To test the validity of the idea, multiple studies have been conducted, ones that show a deficit of mind theory in people with autism (referred to as *mind-blindness*), and ones that attempted to prove that this deficit is independent from mental disability and specific to autism.

Even though mind theory deficits appear – according to studies conducted within this paradigm – in a majority of people with autism, in people with the Asperger syndrome significantly higher occurrence of these results is often observed. According to U. Frith, this phenomenon can be explained in two ways. The first hypothesis assumes that the same basic cognitive deficit is responsible for all autistic spectrum disorders, causing, by appearing in various intensity, both the weaker (the Asperger syndrome) and the stronger consequences (typical, Kanner-type autism). The second hypothesis, one that U. Frith herself leans towards, assumes that the basic cognitive deficit appears with the same level of intensity, but that at one end of the spectrum (including Kanner-style autism) amplifying factors are active, while at the other end (that includes among others the Asperger syndrome) there appear mitigating factors. Among the hypothetical factors that mitigate the primary cognitive deficit in the Asperger syndrome, the author mentions, among others, a sociable temper, a desire to communicate with and belong to the social world, making one undertake often great efforts in order to learn the social code and imitate the behavior of other people (Frith, 2005).

Beside the studies in which authors attempt to determine the ways in which the mind theory deficit manifests itself in people with autism spectrum disorders, and to connect them to the triad of the axial autistic disorders, a number of research projects with a different profile have been undertaken. The second significant type of research within the area of mind theory deficit in autism consists of studies that aim to prove the independence of the mind theory deficit from the occurrence of mental disability, as well as the specificity of mind theory deficit to autism.

The conviction that a single primary cognitive disorder is responsible for the deficits and for the strong extremity of autistic spectrum disorders prompted U. Frith in 1989 to propose a hypothesis that autism is characterized by a specific absence of balance in the integrating of information at different levels. According to the author, the mind theory, although initially promising, cannot explain numerous aspects of autism that do not belong to the triad of axial disorders. Among these aspects are mentioned, among others, a restricted repertoire of interests, obsessive craving of stability (e.g. in the social and physical environ-ment), isolated special skills and savant skills, as well as an interest in parts of objects. Also the results mentioned in the above sub-chapter, which indicated lack of mind theory deficit in some people with autism, suggested further re-search in quest of cognitive deficits underlying autism.

The theory of central coherence can explain, according to U. Frith and F. Happé, the presence of non-triadic aspects of autism. Central coherence refers to the generally appearing tendency towards a synthesis of various information, so as to enable the creation of new complex interpretations and meanings in a specific context, and to leave out less significant details. For example, most people can quite easily summarize a story pointing to its key events and the lead-ing thought, while the recollection of for example the details of an extended description requires more effort (Frith, Happé, 1994; Pisula, 2000)

U. Frith claims that this generally appearing property of information process-ing is disturbed in autism. In her opinion, weak central coherence (or even lack of it) can be responsible for various aspects of autism, in the form of both strong and weak points of cognitive functioning of people with autism. Amidst the strong points in people with autism the author counts, among others, the memory of un-related word strings and objects, shape-based puzzle solving, recognition of verti-cally flipped face images. The weak points include, among others, the memory of sentences and related objects, image-based puzzle solving, recognition of faces (in their typical orientation). U. Frith and F. Happé also recall studies that show how people with autism perform faster and mostly better than control groups in hidden figure test [e.g. CEFT, Children Embedded Figures Test; the Blocks test that belongs to the Wechsler Intelligence Scale (Frith, Happé, 1994)].

It is also significant that U. Frith and F. Happé do not necessarily treat weak central coherence as a deficit, but, taking into account the strong points of people with autism, as a variety of cognitive style, characterized by analytical approach and a focus on details (Frith, Happé, *ibid.*), which signals serious implications for the process of identity research in people with high-functioning autism.

Similar conclusions are presented currently by T. Armstrong, who thinks that in people with autism (in particular with high-functioning autism or the Asperger syndrome) there appears a strong local analysis cognitive style, which favors the exploration of technical and strict fields of study.

F. Levy, while describing a possible reason for the occurrence of weak central coherence, recalls the article "Interacting minds: a biological basis" by C. Frith and U. Frith, in which a hypothesis is put forward that the deficit of central coher-ence appears at an early stage of development of the mind theory, and presents U. Frith's position according to which that deficit is related to a lack of the inte-gration of information from different levels and different perceptional modules.

Cognitive theories of autism enabled a different view on people with autis-tic spectrum disorders. Among the benefits of the cognitive approach U. Frith mentions:

- the creation of a framework that allows to search for factors and mechanisms linking neurological bases with behavioral manifestations;
- differentiation of autism symptoms from additional factors or secondary problems;
- presentation of the huge variety in people with autism, their needs, deficits and skills;
- the start of research on adolescents and adults with autism, and an understanding of the fact that autism is a condition that accompanies an individual throughout their life (Frith, 1994).

Issues of cognitive functioning and the question of identity research in people with the Asperger syndrome or high-functioning autism

One of the premises in approaching the Asperger syndrome (AS) and high-functioning autism (HFA) as two distinct units by the researchers of autism are differences in the areas of verbal communication and cognitive functioning. Studies of the issue do not however produce coherent results that would warrant unequivocal acceptance or rejection of the above thesis. For example, in research conducted by Szatmari et al. a comparison was performed of intelligence profiles, measured with the use of Wechsler Intelligence Scale, between 26 people with AS (average age 14.3 years, average IQ = 86.6) and 17 people with HFA (average age 22.8 years, average IQ = 82.2). Although better results were recorded in the Similarity test in people with AS, in whole test a similar level of performance and similar deficits were found in verbal and non-verbal tests (Koyama et al., 2007). Other results were developed for example in the study by Ozonoff et al., where, analogically, the researchers performed an intelligence profiling using Wechsler Intelligence Scale, in 12 people with AS (average age 13.9 years, average IQ = 115.6) and 23 people with HFA (average age 13.3 years, average IQ = 108.9). People with AS achieved significantly higher results in the Comprehension test, while both groups had substantial problems with the Encoding test (Koyama et al., 2007). Koyama et al. tested 36 people with AS (average age 12.8 years, average IQ = 98.3) and 37 people with HFA (average age 12.6 years, average IQ = 94.6) using Wechsler Intelligence Scale as well as the Tokyo version of CARS (Childhood Autism Rating Scale). People with AS achieved significantly higher verbal IQ and higher results in the Dictionary and Comprehension tests, while people with HFA scored better in the Encoding test. The testing for the symptoms of autism using CARS did not show significant differences between the groups, however, people with AS achieved lower results in the areas of deficits in verbal and non-verbal communication.

A separate issue concerns people with AS or HFA who show intellectual talents and/or isolated special skills of various kinds. They belong to a larger group of talented adolescents with disabilities.

In this context it is worthwhile to recall the concept of identity, proposed by L. Witkowski (1988) and described in the book *Identity and change. An introduction to an epistemological analysis of educational contexts.* It is located in a broad context of reflections on identity, taken up by E. Erikson, J. Habermas and L. Kolberg, and appears very useful for the description of people with high-functioning autism.

As A. Brzezińska writes, giving M. Jarymowicz's idea of identity as an example, the identity of an individual in a psychological approach is formed in two basic dimensions: the personal identity, and the social identity. The personal identity, connected to the formation of the structural "I", "contains individual convictions, interests, needs, motivations, values, way of thinking and valuation criteria" (Brzezińska, 2007, p. 239). In turn, the social identity is connected to the formation of the structural "We", and manifests itself "in the process of the subject's identification with other members of a given social structure, in the experience of ties with them, and in the realization of the community created with other people" (Brzezińska, 2007, p. 239). L. Witkowski decidedly rejects this distinction, claiming that one's own sense of identity (an analogue of personal identity) is to a significant degree constructed socially and built in the process of an individual's exploration of the surrounding socio-cultural reality.

In place of the dual notion of identity, L. Witkowski proposes a triband, horizontal profile of identity, containing the following triad: competence, conception and condition. According to L. Witkowski, "a sense of identity defines an element of human condition (specific-I-in-me), where a sense is for him a state of consciousness prior to knowledge" (Witkowski, 1988, p. 112, author's own translation). A second element of identity is related to the "location" in the world mentioned already above, that is "self-knowledge (specific I-in-world) or a »conception« of one's self" (Witkowski, 1988, p. 112). The process of identity creation has a specific character, because it happens through constant interaction of a human being with their socio-cultural environment, described by L. Witkowski as "contact in action. According to the author of the notion, contact in action is a key issue for the understanding of human identity, because:"

(...) it opens for action a previously indiscernible dimension of competence and creates a new analytical situation. Because, even though a sense of identity is a genetically important part of "I", and from the level of human condition it influences the creation of their conception of self, and affects their mode of presence in the world (contact with it in action), still functional direction of the relation, essential for its understanding, seems to be the opposite. Namely, it can be defined in the form of a "epistemological vector" that expresses the dominant direction of the influence: competence = > conception = > condition (Witkowski, 1988, p. 113, author's own translation).

In Witkowski's opinion, the development of human identity follows from the acquisition (or lack of it) of competence in interactions with other people and elements of the socio-cultural reality, through the formation, on the basis of that competence, of the conception of one's self, to the most narrow level of a sense of one's identity (condition).

Beside the process of identity development described above, according to L. Witkowski, its creation is also influenced by social mechanisms of identity reinforcement. There are three basic types of identification processes that take part in the formation of identity: (1) identification as "recognition" of the environment; (2) identification as "mirroring" of expectations present in the environment, and (3) identification as the process of the development of an ideal "I". The author of the concept notes that the manifestation of a developmental crisis remains dependent on which of the identification processes encounters possible obstacles (Witkowski, 1988, p. 118).

The three bands of identity (competence, conception, condition) overlap the processes of identification. Therefore, identity depends not on the process of identification alone, but rather on the mutual interaction of identification processes.

We propose using Witkowski's triadic concept of identity for descriptions of identity in people with high-functioning autism, assuming that his notion of competence corresponds to their valuation of own social competence, conception – to the subject's self-assessment, and the seeming core of identity, the "condition" – to the concepts of self manifesting itself in auto-narrations of people with autism. This proposition finds an excellent presentation in the theoretical model of a study put forward by P. Pająk (2012) in her unpublished MA thesis, which constitutes an introductory (casuistic) exploration of the analyzed problem, shown in Figure 1.

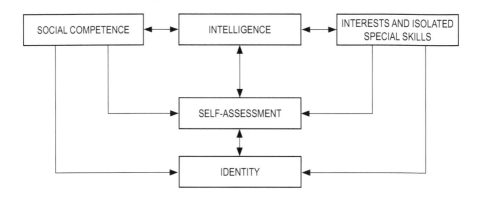

Figure 1. Mutual interactions of the key areas of identity research in people with AS or HFA

Source: own work, after Pająk, 2012

Figure 1 illustrates a hypothetical model of mutual interactions between social competence, intelligence, interests and isolated social skills, and self-assessment, as well as their connection to the process of identity formation.

Social competence and the identity in people with high-functioning autism

As noted by S. Kowalik (2007), the inclusion of the notion of social competence to the discussion of the socialization process allowed one to discern complex relations between an individual in the process of socialization and their social environment. According to A. Matczak, despite the differences between authors in the definition of social competence, one can assume that its is "a disposition that conditions the effectiveness of functioning in social situations" (Matczak, 2001, p. 5). M. Argyle in turn, by social competence understands the "acquisition of skills necessary for achieving desired effects in other people in social situations" (Argyle, 1991, p. 98).

A. Matczak assumes that

> social competence develops as a result of social training, whose intensity depends on personality-temper variables (...), and effectiveness on intelligence, in particular on social intelligence, and emotional intelligence as its constituent (Matczak, 2001, p. 8). Accordingly, she assumes the following definition of social competence, which is the basis of reflections in the current work: social competence (...) is understood as a set of complex skills that condition the effectiveness of performing in specific social situations, and are acquired by an individual in the course of social training (Matczak, 2001, p. 7).

A. Matczak uses the term "competence" in a way that makes it a part of a wider trend in the research on socialization, where authors define it as a set of various skills, not a general capability.

In M. Argyle's opinion, competence as a general capability is not proven, because "a person can perform some tasks better, and other tasks worse" (Argyle, 1991, p. 98). Accordingly, the author assumes that social competence is comprised of various skills, which manifest itself (or not) particularly clearly in the so-called difficult situations. M. Argyle mentions four kinds of such situations:

(1) intimate situations;

(2) situation requiring assertiveness or being the object of attention;

(3) formal (ceremonial) social occasions;

(4) meeting strangers (Argyle, Furnham, Graham, 1982 after: Argyle, 1991).

A. Matczak modified M. Argyle's proposition, putting forward the following classification of diagnostic situations for social competence, together with their descriptions:

(1) intimate situations – close interpersonal contacts, characterized, among others, by significant release of personal information by the partners in the interaction;

(2) situations of social exposition – in which an individual finds themselves in the center of attention of other people, and potentially is subject to an assessment on their part;

(3) formal situations – ones that are governed by strict rules defined within a culture;

(4) situations that require assertiveness – an individual achieves in them their needs or goals by exerting social influence on others, or resisting social influence exerted by them (Matczak, 2001).

From such an approach to social competence, significant implications follow for therapeutic practice carried out for people with AS or HFA. An individual's profile of their social competence can be highly diversified, e.g. problems in situations of social exposition can co-exist with high competence in intimate situations, therefore social skills training should begin with a detailed diagnosis of an individual competence profile.

Despite the fact that the sphere of deficits in social functioning in children with SA/HFA is the object of numerous studies, the area is still poorly understood in the case of adolescents and adults. S.E. Gutstein and T. Whitney (2002) in the paper "Asperger Syndrome and the Development of Social Competence" indicate that they had been able to acquire results from three current studies on this subject. The first of them, conducted by M. Sigman and E. Ruskin (1999) is a longitudinal study of adolescents with HFA, began at pre-school age, which documented lack of improvement in the area of social competence. The second study, conducted by N. Bauminger and C. Kasari in 2000, showed that adolescents with HFA did not understand emotional aspects related to loneliness and friendship, which was not a result of intellectual or linguistic deficits. The researchers decided that it may follow from the specific character of "autistic" friendship, with scant sense of security or companionship, and therefore not reducing the sense of loneliness. In the third study, J. Green, A. Gilchrist, D. Burton and A. Cox (2000) compared adolescents with AS and with severe conduct disorder. The study showed much deeper social deficits in the adolescents with AS, as well as similarly high levels of, among others, anxiety, compulsive-obsessive disorder, depression, and suicidal tendencies in both groups (Gutstein, Whitney, 2002).

An amount of data on the social functioning of adolescents with AS/HFA is provided by research testing the effectiveness of various forms of social training addressed to these groups. Although the initial assessment of social competence before the training is convergent with the results of previously mentioned research, the studies generally report a level of effectiveness of the interventions – it is evidently possible to acquire some social competence in an appropriately structured context (Stitcher et al., 2010; Tse et al., 2007).

In research conducted by Whitehouse et al. on friendship and loneliness in adolescents with AS it was determined that in comparison with the control group, adolescents with AS signaled inferior quality of their closest friendships and less motivation to develop them. Individuals with AS also reported higher indications of loneliness and depression symptoms. The authors indicate that the higher indexes of negative affect can be connected with low quality of social relations, which is often observed in this population.

Self-assessment and identity in people with high-functioning autism

Self-assessment, as noted by B. Ziółkowska (2005), is a property of personality, formed by social interactions, in which an individual builds an image of self.

D. Fecenec mentions two basic sources of self-assessment: observation of own behavior, and feedback from the environment. After E.J. O'Brien and S. Epstein he assumes in turn that the function of self-assessment is to maintain the coherence of the image of Self, which favors the acquisition and integration of new information into this structure, as well as the ordering of experience, hence the coherence of self-assessment is correlated to the coherence of one's identity (Fecenec, 2008).

S. Epstein thinks that the main driver in the creation of the system of self-knowledge is the motivation to avoid averse stimuli and the search for stimuli recognized as pleasurable. Self-assessment develops in the system of Self as a mechanism that regulates the proportions between averse and pleasurable experiences. According to E.J. O'Brien and S. Epstein, self-assessment has a hierarchical construction, which comprises of:

(1) detailed evaluative judgments about self, referring to particular events;

(2) components of self-assessment related o the main areas of human functions: competence, being loved, popularity, self-acceptation, attractiveness, leadership skills, self-control, moral self-acceptance, physical attractiveness, and vitality;

(3) general self-assessment, a most generalized sense of one's value (Fecenec, 2008, pp. 17–19).

Figure 2 shows the hierarchical construction of self-assessment according to E.J. O'Brien and S. Epstein, where GS = General Self-assessment. Accepting the assumption of the hierarchical and complex structure of self-knowledge makes it possible to acquire in research a profile of self-assessment, of diagnostic utility for the sources of low, high, or incoherent self-esteem in adolescents.

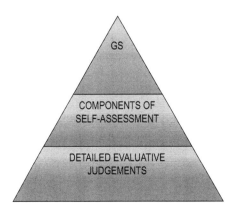

Figure 2. The hierarchical construction of self-assessment

Source: own work, after Fecenec, 2008

Studies of self-assessment in people with the Asperger syndrome are sparse. Therefore, Williamson et al. described their research related to the connection between the level of self-assessment and adjustment in adolescents with AS as an *exploratory study*. It compared a group of 19 adolescents with AS against a group of 19 adolescents from the control group. Four tests were used to determine their attitude towards own competence, social approval, level of anxiety, depression and self-esteem. It turned out that adolescents with AS show a lowered self-esteem, consider themselves as persons less complete in such areas as social skills and sports, and also receive less social approval from their peers (Williamson et al., 2008).

The subject literature also signals divergences between the self-assessment in adolescents with AS/HFA in the area of autistic symptoms and their assessment performed by their parents (Cederlund et al., 2010; Johnson et al., 2009).

Concepts of self and the identity in people with high-functioning autism

For the purposes of identity diagnostics in people with AS or HFA it is postulated to assume that concepts of self constitute a particular element of auto-narration, which is the object of interest for the psychology of narration – one of the currents in the qualitative psychology, connected with hermeneutics. J. Trzebiński notes that narration as understood in this branch of psychology is a particular form of the cognitive representation of reality: "Narrations, that is mental forms of the understanding of the world, assign structure to our experiences in terms of human intentions and problems which result from complications formed during the realization of these intentions" (Trzebiński, 2002, p. 22). A similar function is performed by auto-narrations, but since they refer to one's self, they constitute an important premise for all activities of the subject: "Because an individual takes actions on the basis of what they know about the reality in which they act. The knowledge about self as an active subject of a developing story must b a particularly important premise of that action" (Trzebiński, 2002, p. 38).

A narrative approach seems therefore especially helpful in the examining of people in whom auto-reflection and self-knowledge appear to be for various reasons limited – because of cognitive deficits, or a small amount of social contacts. According to the postulates of L. Wygotski, the application of the narrative approach in the study of the people's concepts of self – including adolescents with the Asperger syndrome and high-functioning autism – could probably help in the uncovering of their sphere of nearest development within this area.

Ending

The progress of the research on the neurobiological conditions of autistic spectrum disorders favors the formulation of numerous questions and points to new perspectives on the describing of autism, unquestioned by most of its renowned theorists. It should be noted, however, that although it remains one of the best investigatively documented issue that confirms the affiliation of autistic spectrum disorders within the category of neurodevelopmental disorders (Penn, 2006), still implications of observed disordsers remain ambiguous. It seems therefore that while engaging in various scientific inspirations, carried out within verified theoretical frameworks, and describing the positive aspects of the autistic spectrum, one should nonetheless contribute to the change of the current social image of autism, and most importantly to minimizing prejudices towards people whose neurological system in certain important areas works differently (cf. Broderick, Ne'eman, 2008).

In order to verify the initial and general diagnostic propositions contained in this article it should be appropriate to apply specific action research. It would cover an initial diagnosis of social competence, self-assessment and resources in adolescents by using self-descriptory techniques (e.g. *The Multidimensional Self-Esteem Inventory* by E.J. O'Brien and S. Epstein as well as two Polish methods, namely: *The Social Competences Questionnaire (Kwestionariusz Kompetencji Społecznych)* by A. Matczak and the *Multidimensional Questionnaire of Preferences (Wielowymiarowy Kwestionariusz Preferencji)* by A. Matczak, A. Jaworowska, A. Ciechanowicz, E. Zalewska and J. Stańczak. Furthermore, two qualitative methods were applied: *Test 'I am'* by P.G. Zimbardo used the in-depth diagnostic interview with the adolescent and their significant others as a narrative technique, and an unstructured interview with a standardized list of questions with reference to interests and self-concepts, as well as a narrative interview (pre-test), the psychological intervention in the form of social training combined with relaxation training, and then a renewed diagnosis performed in order to assess the effectiveness of the intervention (post-test).

References

Argyle, M. (1991). *Psychologia stosunków międzyludzkich*, Warszawa: Wydawnictwo Naukowe PWN.

Attwood, T. (2006). *Zespół Aspergera. Wprowadzenie.* Poznań: Zysk i S-ka Wydawnictwo.

Baron-Cohen, S., Frith, U., Leslie, A.M. (1985). Does the autistic child have a „theory of mind?", *Cognition*, Vol. 21, 37–46.

Baron-Cohen, S., Hadwin, J., Hollin, P. (2010). *Jak uczyć dzieci z autyzmem czytania umysłu.* Kraków: Wydawnictwo JAK.

Broderick, A.A., Ne'eman, A. (2008). Autism as metaphor: narrative and counter narrative. *International Journal of Inclusive Education*, 5–6 (12), 459–476.

Brzezińska, A. (2007). *Społeczna psychologia rozwoju.* Warszawa: Wydawnictwo Naukowe „Scholar".

Cederlund, M., Hagberg, B., Gillberg, C. (2010). Asperger syndrome in adolescent and young adult males. Interview, self- and parent assessment of social, emotional, and cognitive problems. *Research In Developmental Disabilities*, 31(2), 287–298.

Craig, A.O., Bond, L., Burns, J.M., Vella-Brodrick, D.A., Sawyer, S.M. (2003). Adolescent resilience: a concept analysis. *Journal of adolescence*, 26, 1–11.

Crocker, J., Quinn, D. (2008). *Piętno społeczne i Ja: znaczenia, sytuacje i samoocena.* [W:] T.F. Heatherton, R.E. Kleck, M.R. Hebl, J.G. Hull (red.). *Społeczna psychologia piętna*, 149–174. Warszawa: Wydawnictwo Naukowe PWN.

Fecenec, D. (2008). *Wielowymiarowy Kwestionariusz Samooceny MSEI. Polska adaptacja. Podręcznik.* Warszawa: Pracownia Testów Psychologicznych.

Frith, U. (red.) (2005). *Autyzm i zespół Aspergera.* Warszawa: Państwowy Zakład Wydawnictw Lekarskich.

Frith, U., Happé, F. (1994). Autism: beyond 'theory of mind.' *Cognition*, 50, 115–132.

Gillberg, C. (2005). *Kliniczne i neurobiologiczne aspekty zespołu Aspergera na podstawie sześciu badań rodzin.* [W:] U. Frith (red.). *Autyzm i zespół Aspergera*, 150–179. Warszawa: Państwowy Zakład Wydawnictw Lekarskich,.

Greenberg, M.T. (2006). Promoting resilience in children and youth. Preventive intervention and their interface with neuroscience. *Annals of the New York Academy of Sciences*, Vol. 1094, Resilience in Children, 139–150.

Gutstein, S.E., Whitney, T. (2002). Asperger Syndrome and the Development of Social Competence. *Focus On Autism and Other Developmental Disabilities Journal*, 17(3), 161.

Johnson, S.A., Filliter, J.H., Murphy, R.R. (2009). Discrepancies Between Self- and Parent-Perceptions of Autistic Traits and Empathy in High Functioning Children and Adolescents on the Autism Spectrum. *Journal of Autism and Developmental Disorders*, 39(12), 1706–1714.

Kumpfer, K.L., Summerhays, J.F. (2006). Prevention Approaches to Enhance Resilience among High-Risk Youth. Comments on the Papers of Dishion, Connell and

Greenberg. *Annals of the New York Academy of Sciences*, Vol. 1094, Resilience in Children, 151–163.

Kowalik, S. (2007). *Psychologia rehabilitacji*, Warszawa: WAIP.

Koyama, T., Tachimori, H., Osada, H., Takeda, T., Kurita, H. (2007). Cognitive and symptom profiles in Asperger's syndrome and high-functioning autism. *Psychiatry, Clinical Neurosciences*, 61(1), 99–104.

Leslie, A.M. (1987). Pretense and Representation: The Origins of "Theory of Mind." *Psychological Review*, 94 (4), 412–426.

Leslie, A.M. (1992). Pretense, Autism, and the Theory-of-Mind Module. *Current Directions in Psychological Science* (Wiley-Blackwell), 1(1), 18–21.

Luthar, S.S., Zelazo, L.B. (2003). *Research on Resilience. An Integrative Review*. [In:] Luthar, S.S. (Ed.). *Resilience and Vulnerability* (510–549). Cambridge: Cambridge University Press.

Luthar, S.S. (2006). *Resilience in development: A synthesis of research across five decades*. [In:] D. Cicchetti, D.J. Cohen (Eds.). *Developmenthal Psychopatology: Risk, disorder, and adaptation*, Vol. 3, (740–795). New York: Wiley.

Matczak, A. (2001). *Kwestionariusz Kompetencji Społecznych. Podręcznik*. Warszawa: Pracownia Testów Psychologicznych.

Pająk, P. (2012). *Kompetencje społeczne, inteligencja oraz zainteresowania, a tożsamość adolescentów z zespołem Aspergera i wysokofunkcjonującym autyzmem*. Niepublikowana praca magisterska. Kraków: Archiwum Instytutu Psychologii Stosowanej UJ.

Penn, H. (2006). Neurobiological correlates of autism: a review of recent research. *Child Neuropsychology: A Journal On Normal And Abnormal Development In Childhood And Adolescence*, 12(1), 57–79.

Pisula, E. (2000). *Autyzm u dzieci. Diagnoza, klasyfikacja, etiologia*. Warszawa: Wydawnictwo Naukowe PWN.

Sameroff, A., Rosenblum, K. (2006). Psychosocial Constraints on the Development of Resilience. *Annals of the New York Academy of Sciences*, Vol. 1094, Resilience in Children, 116–124.

Shtayermman, O. (2007). Peer Victimization in Adolescents and Young Adults Diagnosed with Asperger's Syndrome: A Link to Depressive Symptomatology, Anxiety Symptomatology and Suicidal Ideation. *Issues in Comprehensive Pediatric Nursing*, 30(3), 87–107.

Shtayermman, O. (2009). An Exploratory Study of the Stigma Associated With a Diagnosis of Asperger's Syndrome: The Mental Health Impact on the Adolescents and Young Adults Diagnosed With a Disability With a Social Nature. *Journal of Human Behavior in the Social Environment*, 19 (3), 298–313.

Stichter, J.P., Herzog, M.J., Visovsky, K., Schmidt, C., Randolph, J., Schultz, T. (2010). Social Competence Intervention for Youth with Asperger Syndrome and High-functioning Autism: An Initial Investigation. *Journal of Autism, Developmental Disorders*, 40(9), 1067–1079.

Szatmari, P. (2000). The Classification of Autism, Asperger's Syndrome, and Pervasive Developmental Disorder. *Canadian Journal of Psychiatry*, 45(8), 731.

Talarowska, M., Florkowski, A., Gałecki, P., Zboralski, K. (2010). *Psychologiczne koncepcje rozwoju autyzmu*. [W:] T. Pietras, A. Witusik, P. Gałecki (red.). *Autyzm – epidemiologia, diagnoza i terapia*. 99–118. Wrocław: Wydawnictwo Continuo.

Trzebiński, J. (2002). *Narracyjne konstruowanie rzeczywistości.* [W:] J. Trzebiński (red.). *Narracja jako sposób rozumienia świata,* (17–42). Gdańsk: Gdańskie Wydawnictwo Psychologiczne.

Tse, J., Strulovitch, J., Tagalakis, V., Linyan, M., Fombonne, E. (2007). Social Skills Training for Adolescents with Asperger Syndrome and High-Functioning Autism. *Journal of Autism and Developmental Disorders,* 37(10), 1960–1968.

Williamson, S., Craig, J., Slinger, R. (2008). Exploring the relationship between measures of self-esteem and psychological adjustment among adolescents with Asperger syndrome. *Autism,* 14(4), 391–402.

Witkowski, L. (1988). *Tożsamość i zmiana. Wstęp do epistemologicznej analizy kontekstów edukacyjnych.* Toruń: Wydawnictwo Naukowe Uniwersytet Mikołaja Kopernika.

Yates, T.M., Egeland, B., Sroufe, A. (2003). *Rethinking* resilience. *A developmental process perspective.* [In:] S.S. Luthar (Ed.). *Resilience and Vulnerability* (243–259). Cambridge: Cambridge University Press.

Ziółkowska, B. (2005), *Okres dorastania. Jak rozpoznać ryzyko i jak pomagać?* [W:] A. Brzezińska (red.). *Psychologiczne portrety człowieka. Praktyczna psychologia rozwojowa.* (379–422). Gdańsk: Gdańskie Wydawnictwo Psychologiczne.

Urszula Tokarska

Pedagogical University, Cracow

"THE BENEFICIAL LIFE STORIES." HEALTH AND MENTAL RESILIENCE FROM THE NARRATIVE PERSPECTIVE

Abstract

The article aims to explore the narrative dimension of mental health and resilience. Empirically proven, the high adaptation value of the narrative structuring of individual experience is considered in the context of the relational health model based on the discursive approach. It encompasses a healthy and functioning adult personality as a complex model organising the diversity of individual experience (polyphonic structure) that emerges above the level of "subjective positions" in which individuals experience the world and themselves. In such an approach, the ability to transcend a one-sided point of view and the capacity for dialogue between various perspectives are the key to the mental health and resilience of individuals. This dynamic process derives from the formal and content characteristics of "self-narratives" created by individuals as well as the rules according to which they are combined into comprehensive life stories through narrative identity.

The description of the indicators of what is known as a "good/healthy self-narrative" that are presented in relevant literature and the overview of the essence of positive influence exerted in the process of creating a self-narrative (that ultimately have an impact on its "beneficial" nature) form a basis for defining "narrative preventive factors." They can be used to design projects that aim at the *narrative promotion of mental health and resilience*. It is advisable that such projects additionally take into account the existential issues in the professional work that enhances the narrative structuring of individual experience. Is appears that they can be carried out at all life stages and, at the same time, consider individual and currently available levels in the development of their recipients and their self-narratives.

Key words: narrative approach in psychology, resilience, dialogical dimension of personality

Introduction

Psychologists commonly agree that the entirety of *events* in one's biography does not constitute one's *life* as long as the selected ones (observed, interpreted and remembered) are not transformed into individual *experience*. "Narrative-oriented" psychologists add that certain experiences can take a form of re-counted episodes and subsequently be combined into a comprehensive *auto-biographic narrative*. The point at which life meets narrative is regulated by narrative identity, a superordinate semantic structure that shapes the way in which meaningful events are organised into a coherent autobiographic narrative (Dryll, 2010). The narrative structure of experience serves as "recipes for struc-turing experience" (Bruner, 1990) that "make a coherent whole of what we do and experience" (Śleszyński, 1998), thus defining the meaning of both particular experiences and individual biographies in their entirety. The empirically proven beneficial potential of narrative thinking (in contrast to the paradigmatic mode of processing information, Bruner, 1986) is conducive to the mental health and well-being of individuals (Pennebaker, Chung, 2007) and, according to some researchers, it even constitutes their necessary condition (Salvatore, Dimaggio, Semenari, 2004; Stemplewska-Żakowicz, Zalewski, 2010). The narrative inter-pretation of events in many respects proves beneficial to the healthy function-ing of individuals and is correlated with such dimensions as an enhanced sense of control over events, higher will and motivation levels, more frequent sense of tranquillity, better identification with other human beings that in turn leads to an increase in empathy and readiness to help others (Trzebiński, 2005). This paper focusses on the relation between the narrative mode of processing information and mental health and resilience in the face of difficult situations, the latter being defined as "(…) unexpected adaptation in the face of serious adversity allow-ing to maintain or subsequently achieve a positive developmental trajectory" (Hauser, Allen, 2007, p. 567).

Regarded as beneficial to individual health, a multi-layered, coherent and meaningful "well-developed and peaceful life narrative" is characterised by a particular structure and complexity as well as content. Such a story should pro-vide its narrator with a sense of continuity, individual experience and self-agency and, at the same time, should remain understandable for others. The change of the narrative position of the subject, which leads from a domination of the ex-ternal perspective through internal to the transcendent one (Straś-Romanowska, 2005a), is considered one of the leading manifestations of its beneficial nature. It is assumed that the change that emerges through numerous "shifts" between various positions, or voices, of the subject which in turn should optimally result in achieving the state of "internal democracy" (Stemplewska-Żakowicz, 2002) constitutes both the condition for and the manifestation of complete (i.e. rela-tional) mental health.

The article defines mental health and resilience in the face of difficult situations both with reference to life-long personal development and including the individual existential adaptation perspective (Straś-Romanowska, 2005b; Tokarska, 2004, 2006, 2009). For this reason, together with the multi-faceted description of narrative structuring and integration, it emphasises the significance of not only *how* the individually created autobiographic narratives present their content, but also *what* they are about. The description of the assumptions of relational and polyphonic dimension of health in the discursive approach, empirical and clinical criteria for a "good narrative" and detailed characteristics of self-narratives that have an impact on its "beneficial" potential allow us to define the individual approach to the narrative promotion of mental health and resilience. The impact proposed takes into account the narrative needs and tasks, which evolve in the course of individual life, and the methods that help to meet these needs stem from the narrative approach to psychology. It appears to be useful both on the level of the leading metaphor of "life story" which provides the context for the process of understanding others and as a set of proposals for specific methods to make a practical impact. The main context in this respect is provided by theoretical anthropology that defines a human being as a creature whose developmental tasks are limited neither to survival and social adaptation nor self-actualisation proposed by humanistic psychology and which aim to transcend individual psyche (Łoś, 2010; Straś-Romanowska, 2005b).

The relational and polyphonic dimension of health in the discursive approach

The relational and polyphonic dimension of health in the discursive approach refers to the narrative understanding of ego structure and is based on the argument that mental health relies on integration. In order to create a "coherent, well-developed and peaceful" life narrative (synonymous with mental health), it is necessary to achieve subsequent levels in the development of self-narrative, which are conditioned by the interaction between various social, cultural and individual factors.

Mental health as dependent on integration

The discursive mind model (Stemplewska-Żakowicz, 2001, 2002; Hermans, 1999; Hermans, Kempen, 1993) propounds that telling a story does not take place only in the "interpersonal" space, but also in the "intrapersonal" one (Stemplewska-Żakowicz, 2004; Soroko, 2008). Formulated in the human mind, the potential "points of view" that stem from internalised values and cultural patterns, social principles and scripts and numerous individual influences translate into numerous subjective positions or voices (*polyphony*).

Their interaction is referred to as dialogism and the voices that emerge in the process create a self-narrative (Botella, Herrero, 2000). In the discursive approach, individual personality constitutes a structure that emerges above the level of particular "subjective positions" as a complex model that integrates the relations between them, while the capacity for dialogue, i.e. the ability to transcend a one-side point of view, is the key to the healthy functioning of individuals. "In the light of the dialogic approach, mental health turns out not to be anchored in the unity of personality, but in its multitude, in diversity capable of dialogue (Stemplewska, 2002, 110; translated by the author). Such an understanding of the issue leads to a new and general, "relational" pattern of mental health. Since numerous voices coexist in the human mind and the discursive self is polyphonic by nature, the optimum functioning of individuals is dependent on the state of "internal democracy" that may be established between particular subjective positions. Consequently, narratives that emerge on various levels and in various relational contexts will remain in dynamic interaction, thus both enabling the integration of personality and maintaining its diversity. The protection of the narratively-defined mental health, well-being and resilience in turn consists in the intentional and narrative facilitation of communication between internalised subjective positions, according to the assumption adopted by Bruner (1990) that "self is a perpetually rewritten story."

The narrative structure of self

Introduced into narrative psychology by Sarbin (1986), the concept of the „narrative structure of self" draws upon the distinction between the I and the Me proposed by W. James (and subsequently by G. Mead). The I is the author, the Me in turn is the agent or the lyrical persona. The I creates a story with the Me as its character. Such narrative construction constitutes a mode that organises events, actions and descriptions of events (Sarbin, 1986, as cited [In:] Neckar, 2000; Tokarska, 1994). Hermans (1996) adds that narratives combine elements derived from both the perception of reality and imagination and that telling a story assumes the presence of both real and imaginary dialogues. Hermans propounds that events in narratives are organised in a spatial-temporal manner and that narratives concentrate on their main characters. When making an attempt to define the leading universal themes that explain the composition of a story and its connections with the patters on the individual level, Hermans created the concept of "self as an organised process of valuation" (Hermans, Hermans-Jansen, 1995; Neckar, 2000). This approach understands the "dialogic self" as an imaginary space that spans between various positions and is endowed with the capacity to move between them. Thus, the complexity of self is composed of various voices that are involved in dialogue and tell stories to each other. As a result, it is possible to combine individual temporal dimensions and such diverse components as the real, the ideal or the necessary. The interesting interpretation of the concept of self was provided by approaches that take advantage of contemporary cognitive and neurobiological views on processing information in the mind (Cozolino, 2004; Salvatore et al., 2004). One such interpretation was proposed by D. Denett (1992), who describes self as a central character in an autobiography which acts as an important and, at the same time, fictional focus of attention and establishes equilibrium between fragmentary voices and the self-narratives they create.

A coherent life narrative

A better, more coherent and more narratively structured story, known as a "peaceful life narrative" (Siegel, 2011) is created through narrative structuring that integrates separate elements into a more coherent representation. In optimum conditions, such a representation develops gradually and allows achieving subsequent levels of narrative complexity (see Salvatore et al., 2004). Acquired in infancy and early childhood, the early behavioural patterns are strengthened as characteristic qualities of the mind at later stages of individual life. According to Siegel, the way in which the mind develops at the earliest stages of its development depends on the attachment styles (secure, avoidant, ambivalent/resistant and disorganised) created through interaction with significant persons. They will later influence the ways in which individual life narratives are created that either improve or affect the functioning of individuals. The adaptation narrative about one's own existence stands a better chance to emerge naturally in those adults whose biographies are dominated by a "(…) peaceful relationship between parents and their children that fosters the development of the commissural fibres in the central pre-frontal part of children's brains" (Siegel, 2011, p. 229).

People that construct „peaceful life stories" are able to speak about their past in a more detached manner, thus finding a balance between positive and negative influences; and can also oscillate between memories and reflection on these memories and discern how their self-understanding and development evolve over time. Their stories combine a large number of distinctive details that allow the listeners to understand them in their entirety. Self narratives that are referred to as belittling, self-absorbed or indecisive can in turn cause difficulties or have a disturbing effect. The characteristic feature of the *belittling* narrative is its incoherence, or "blank spaces in the story:" no recollection of the details concerning the past relationships with others and the declaration that the past has no impact on the present. The identity that emerges as a result is autonomous by nature while its central theme concentrates on the solitary struggle with life. As regards the content, such a story does not attach importance to relationships with others, and as regards its formal features, it is very succinct. The *self-absorbed narrative* is incoherent in a different way: themes that are anchored in the past burst into present experiences of the individual, which makes it difficult for them to make the most of their current situation. Siegel attaches the most negative potential in this respect to the *indecisive narrative*, which is also referred to as "disorganised" or "disturbed." The narrator temporarily breaks off narration (see the concept of "breaking the thread of the narrative by suffering" by Ricoeur, 1992), thus experiencing their own past again, in return for the story, as it were. The concealed suffering together with a state of intellectual dissociation revives and begins to override the actual experience ("unhealed trauma or resentment that exist in the mind bring about a narrative which is prone to confusion and disorder at those moments when trauma or loss resurface in the mind, (…) a generally coherent story may become fragmented (…) and lead to disintegration") (Siegel, 2011, p. 250).

A developed peaceful life narrative

Depending on the kind and degree of possible disturbances in the construction of individual self-narratives (self-narratives that are incomplete, chaotic, repetitive, with a tragic ending, etc.), it may turn out to be necessary to take action to make them more adaptive. The common way to provide assistance in this respect is to use the narrative function of the mind, which allows for the absent themes in the story to emerge and makes it possible to fill in the missing components and study the links between the experiences that occur in separate temporal dimensions. At its best, the "new narrative integration" allows one to create a "developed peaceful life story," which, even though previously unavailable to the individual, opens up the chance to enhance their current self-awareness levels and discover a more comprehensive "understanding of their life." Some people may fail to "reconstruct" their autobiographic childhood memories, also because they may have never occurred in the early, pre-narrative stages in the development of their self-narratives.

Levels in the development of self-narratives

In the model of the development of self-narratives proposed by Salvatore et al. (2004) the three out of five levels in the narrative structuring of experience (pre-narrative, proto-narrative and unconscious procedural) remain decidedly beyond the individual's insight and interference. It is only by achieving the level of conscious symbolic narrative (closely connected to latent narrative from previous stages) that one can "(…) freely access the events remembered in the past and the vision of possible future. The existing scripts of the individual and others allow the individual to formulate conscious expectations of what the interaction with others should be like (…). The content that emerges on the level of symbolic narrative may be consciously reflected on and modified." According to the model, the fifth level, which is also known as verbal interactive narrative, is the most advanced and allows for complex narratives to emerge through both internal dialogue and dialogue with others. As they combine various points of view into a coherent and dynamic whole, individuals may consciously modify, reconstruct and complete their self-narratives. This facilitates the integration of identity and personality development and is felt by individuals as "using their own experience." Subsequent potential levels in the development of narrative and its complexity are not achieved automatically and may require external assistance.

The concept of emotional markers that attach *meaning* to the early autobiographic experiences of individuals (Stemplewska-Żakowicz, Zalewski, 2010) appear to be a significant factor that may be conducive to a better understanding of possible difficulties that occur in the development of a coherent life narrative. These markers allow individuals to relate the sensations of the body to the changes in their environment through micro-episodes and micro-scenarios which are indispensable in the process of creating coherent behavioural scripts characteristic of the later stages in their development and which lead to the creation of coherent and healthy narratives. It is the possibility of reaching primordial bodily experience and its subsequent symbolisation that makes these narratives more fluent and personally experienced (Richert, 2003), thus making an impact on the process of either *healthy or disturbed meaning-making* (Greenberg, Angus, 2004). The larger the distance between life stories and the bodily experience of their narrators, the more likely it is that they will experience suffering.

Empirical and clinical criteria for a "good narrative"

The question that this article primary aims to answer is what makes the narrative understanding of one's life meet the criteria for a "good narrative" and what specific qualities of self-narratives are conducive to their beneficial nature. This remains in line with the assumption, based on empirical research and clinical observations, that not every "good" self-narrative is a „beneficial self-narrative" by default. The basic methods of collecting data to formulate these indicators derive from the clinical analysis of dysfunctional narratives (characteristic of patients that are schizophrenic, paranoid or dissociated after traumatic experiences). The analysis of therapeutic narrative processes (talking cure) that aim to restore the healthy functioning of disturbed self-narratives provides a set of interesting interpretations in this respect. Obviously, one has to mention the commonly discussed results of the empirical research on the health-promoting impact of the narrative structuring of experience stimulated through expressive writing (writing cure). In the recent years, it seems especially popular to study the issue of pro-developmental effects of the narrative structuring of experiences that are highly emotionally charged and lead to posttraumatic growth. The shift in interest from mental health to resilience in turn leads to a more detailed study of self-narratives created by individuals with higher resilience levels. The analyses of key and, at the same time, recurring elements in their life stories ("resilience key stories") provide a valuable material in the process of identifying *preventive factors* that may be later taken into account when designing therapeutic and preventive activities (Hauser, Allen, 2006, 2007).

The clinical analysis of dysfunctional narratives

The act of "subverting" the knowledge we have on dysfunctional narratives is the simplest way to identify the health-promoting narratives in individual experience. The difficulty to articulate their own story by individuals who have no clinically diagnosed disturbances and whose stories have certain gaps, blank spaces or asymmetries may manifest its consequences on many levels. The disturbances observed in the functioning of their memory are interpreted as an effect of failure to coordinate complementary memory systems, declarative and non-declarative. It can also be observed that they find it difficult to make a decision and solve everyday tasks, have lower motivation levels to act in a long term perspective and have difficulty planning their future (Trzebiński, 2002).

However, it is the analysis of self-narratives created by patients with specific clinically diagnosed disturbances (known as *illness narratives*, Kleinmann, 1988) that provide the data which ultimately proves the beneficial effect that life stories have on the mental health of individuals. Researchers that describe the content and weaker structuring of life stories created by patients with schizophrenia (Lysaker, Lysaker, 2001, 2006) came to the conclusion that they can be identified by the disturbed structure of their stories, most frequently manifested by two phenomena: *cacophony* and *monologue*. *Cacophony* takes place when many equivalent self-narratives make an attempt to emerge simultaneously, without any structuring or hierarchy. A disturbed monologue in turn occurs when comprehensive overriding (dominant) narratives (monologues) emerge in a sequence, one by one and yet with no relation to each other. Lysakers (2003a, 2003b) also mention the following characteristic features of schizoid self-narratives: no subjective character or narrator in the story and the narrator rarely relating the story to its audience.

The clinically recognisable features of paranoid narratives can in turn be found in a story that attaches a peculiar meanings to the individual's experiences by creating a strongly and unequivocally polarised sense of good and evil, expressing a conviction impending doom and presenting the self as completely separated from the internal states experience by others (Keen, 1986). Nochi (1998) studied dysfunctional narratives created by people with posttraumatic brain damage. After the traumatic event they had experienced, the majority of his patients were not able to construct a coherent self-narrative or find continuity between their behaviours prior to the damage and after it. This state was closely correlated with a deep sense of confusion, which they recounted as a "loss of self." The therapy they underwent relieved the majority of the patients as they could restore continuity, coherence and meaning to their lives. Gazzaniga (as cited [In:] Denet, 1992) claims that individuals with a dissociated brain have a peculiar talent to unify their experience, which is considerably disjointed. "There is a likelihood that this tendency is not only due to their specific situations, but it also reveals a more general trend, typical of all individuals, to create stories that unifies our experience and makes it more coherent" (Denett, 1992, as cited [In:] Neckar, 2000, p. 140). Dimaggio and Semenari (2001) also propounded a unique classification of the most frequent dysfunctional narratives, which allows the identification of the traits that are typical of particular mental disorders. According to researchers, they include impoverished narratives that emerge as a result of the inappropriate emotional marking of early individual experiences or because of the cognitively restrictive educational environment; as well as disoriented (confused) and poorly integrated narratives. Poorly integrated narratives may encompass stories that fail to integrate self-representations with representations of others or to structure fragmentary self-narratives (Chrzczonowicz, 2011).

The analysis of the essence of narrative therapeutic processes

From the narrative point of view, the mental well-being of individuals constitutes the quality of their self-stories and is particularly instrumental in the process of piecing together the three elements of its multi-layered structure (Soroko, 2008). They belong to the level of social and cultural discourse, personal experiences and narrative structuring of experience. While cultural discourse is present in individual (raw) experience, the final shape of the story depends on narrative structuring (construction and interpretation). Problems arise when the content of socially and culturally influenced narratives is not in line with the narrator's preferences. As some stories are socially and culturally privileged over other stories, "(…) people fail to construct stories they prefer and construct stories they are doomed to" (Soroko, 2008, p. 96) and local or individual stories lose the "power to create reality," which in turn is manifested by "narrative asymmetries" (Ochs, Capps, 1996, see also the concept of *culture and social ecology in promoting resilience among populations*, Ungar, 2012).

Sequences of changes in the way individual experience is narrated by clients in the process of therapy are referred to as the narrative process (Soroko, 2008). In the classical narrative therapy (Morgan, 2000; White, Epston, 1990; White, Denborought, 1999), this leads towards creating an alternative story by the client (alternative to the previously dominant problem narrative). In therapies that draw on the model of the discursive mind, the narrative process aims to facilitate communication between internalised subjective positions. In the humanistic-existential approach to narrative therapy (Richert, 2002, 2003), it in turn aims to justify the choice of an alternative narrative in a symbolised experience of the body (felt sense). In the classical narrative therapy, the work on an alternative story begins at the stage of cognitive externalisation of the problem together with seeking unique outcomes in which the individual did not experience the problem or coped with it well. Subsequent stages focus on strengthening a new positive theme and make an attempt to formulate a self-narrative which presents the client, and the character in the narrative, as stronger (in the present and in the future) than the problem he or she encounters. At the same time, it is assumed that emerging alternative self-narratives stand a better chance to structure the experience of their authors when they are presented to the outsider witness group. Therapeutic achievements are in principle documented and celebrated, often with literary means such as certificates or letters, and they are also circulated as concrete examples (details of the client provided with the client's approval) of bring-it-back-practices. Subsequent stages of the therapeutic process are enhanced with various additional narrative techniques (metaphors such as "life as a book" or "life as a journey") and narrative texts that draw upon cultural legacy and encourage to test the alternative ways to arrive at self-understanding (Tokarska, 1995, 2008a). Mechanisms used in narrative therapy to construct an alternative and health-promoting self-narrative (see Tokarska, 2002) reorganise the system of memory that stimulates narrative memory and distance individuals from their own experiences, including difficult situations. While the symbolic and universal transformation of experience ("what universal sense does my story have?") plays a logotherapeutic role ("what can I learn from my own story?"), the multilevel narrative integration of life experiences becomes a basis for a narrative identity. Therapists act as "privileged listeners" and their feedback also has an impact on further modifications to the narrative process. Since it is assumed in narrative therapies that narratives do not represent an identity, problems or life in general, but constitute an identity, problems and life (Carr, 1998), by creating "alternative stories" individuals can open new possibilities in structuring their own lives. The aim of therapy is to strengthen the client's sense of agency (authorship) and co-author their alternative stories so that their impact on the client's life is more powerful than that of problem narratives. The crux of the change is in reorganising the client's indentity (around alternative self-narratives) and facilitating the process of identification with alternative narratives that replace the previously dominating problem narratives (see Soroko, 2008; Tokarska, 2000a; 2000b).

It is worth noticing that, in narrative therapy, the direction of proposed activities is reverted (when compared with other types of therapy) and founded on the philosophical and linguistic assumption that speech can influence thought processes. If we assume that "speech can influence thought" (according to the concept of "speech as a gesture" and contrary to the understanding of "speech as a sign," see Merleau-Ponty), the patient's narrative may become not only an "effect and touchstone, but also a tool for change" (Grzegorek, 2005, p. 121). Such an effect can be achieved if we introduce new communication patterns, give up dysfunctional speaking habits and eliminate infelicitous phrasing or even whole narrative structures.

The empirical study of the health-promoting role of expressive writing

Numerous experiments on expressive writing support the thesis that narratives on emotionally significant events have an impact on the mental and social well-being of individuals and can be treated as a "writing cure," which is similar to a "talking cure (Lepore, Smyth, 2002). The relevant study results demonstrate that those individuals who describe their significant emotional and personal experiences enjoy better health, which can be seen both in terms of their self-descriptive, physiological and behavioural indicators and, for example, in the decreasing number of their medical appointments (Baikie, Wilhelm, 2005; Campbell, Pennebaker, 2003; Kaufman, Sexton, 2006; Lyubomirsky et al., 2006; Pennebaker, Seagal, 1999; Pennebaker, Chung, 2007; Soroko, 2012; Stiles et al., 1999). This corresponds with the assumptions of narrative therapies that propound the necessity to find a narrative which allows individuals to understand, assimilate and overcome the effect of their traumatic experiences (or other powerful emotional experiences). This phenomenon is particularly visible as *post-traumatic growth* (Błaszczak, 2002; Denham, 2008; Juczyński, 2012; Mansfield et al., 2010; Kubacka-Jasiecka, Kuleta, 2012).

The researchers of expressive writing (Pennebaker, 1997) describe the essence of the positive impact in the process of constructing a narrative both as a disclosure, even if only to oneself, of difficult experiences and as a change in the way highly emotionally charged experiences are encoded as they are transformed into words (code-switching, from analogue to digital). However, the majority of relevant research proves that it is only by creating descriptions that develop into increasingly structured narratives that individuals can benefit from the process of therapy. "A mere verbal expression of difficult emotional content is not therapeutic; it is only through narrative structuring that one can benefit from the healing powers of such an expression" (Stemplewska-Żakowicz, Zalewski, 2010, p. 21).

Characteristic features of self-narratives created by highly resilient individuals

The research on self-narratives created by individuals with higher-than-average-resilience levels provides interesting data on the indicators of health-promoting life narratives. The analyses of resilience key stories are carried out in various research contexts, the most interesting of which seem to be longitudinal study projects. One of the most developed (lasting for two decades) studies on resilience that used narrative material was carried out by Hauser and Allen (2007). In their study carried out in 1980s, the study group composed of teenagers who had experienced several concurrent significant life difficulties (spent time in metal hospital and were diagnosed as socially maladjusted) gave detailed answers in an open narrative survey. After many years, as the study group members started to live their adult lives in various social contexts, the surveys were analysed again. The majority of the study group members were diagnosed again using standardised clinical tools and new autobiographic surveys in terms of the degree and quality of the way in which they overcame their previous and current life difficulties. Resilience narrative preventive factors were identified on the basis of the comparative analysis of the self-narratives created during their adolescence and adulthood. As a result, key structural and content patterns that organise both adolescent and adult self-narratives turned out to be considerably stable.

Formally speaking, Hauser and Allen regard complexity and coherence as specific factors that differentiate the way in which individuals resilient to serious life difficulties structure their experience (as compared with individuals that have low resilience levels). However, as far as the content of resilience narratives is concerned, they point to the specific and repetitive pattern of self-representations and representations of interpersonal relations. They claim that resilience representations imply a sense of agency and growing self-awareness levels concerning both emotional and mental states. This is manifested not only when individuals undertake specific actions, but also by active decision-making that helps them to take care of themselves when repeatedly faced with life difficulties. This aspect corresponds with the notion of a complete self-narrative structure, which in turn implies a conscious and proactive approach to potential obstacles (both in the context of "life philosophy" that accepts such a state of affairs and a set of skills and tools that help to overcome life difficulties). The resilience narratives also contain descriptions of conscious decision-making processes that lead to realising individual intentions and include procedures that help materialise ideas. The self-image of their narrators offers numerous examples of their perseverance and ambition. The analyses of self-narratives show that their narrators assess themselves is a realistic manner and have a highly complex sense of self. Their representations of interpersonal relations in turn reflect on the motives behind other people's actions, attach high importance to close friendship and demonstrate a proactive approach when establishing and maintaining other interpersonal relations. Present in their current narratives, the elements of previous narratives (later assessed by researchers as conducive to resilience) also contained self-described changes.

Detailed characteristics of self-narratives that influence their "beneficial" nature

The detailed characteristics of self-narratives that influence their "beneficial" nature can be split into two basic sets of factors: the degree of their narrative structuring (complexity, coherence) and their content.

A complete self-narrative pattern and self-narrative style

Psychology defines narrative not only as a particular form of verbal expression, but also as a form of knowledge, which may not be realised by its subject. By contrast to verbal narratives, this constitutes a "narrative in action," a manifestation of an automatic and unconscious understanding of events (Dryll, 2010; Stemplewska-Żakowicz, Zalewski, 2010; Trzebiński, 2002). Such an understanding is regulated by means of cognitive self-narrative patterns, whose components include the following: a character with a repertory of his/her potential intentions, plans and obstacles expected to emerge in the process as well as circumstances, opportunities and specific ways of coping with difficulties (Trzebiński, 2002). The degree to which a given unit of a narrative pattern is complete and logical influences the way in which has an impact on whether it is effective in selected areas of the functioning of individuals. For example, if an image of self (narrator) has not been clearly articulated as a character in a story, this may be treated as a manifest of a secondary condition for a variety of disturbances that affect the individual's self-awareness and self-knowledge and the possibility of being understood by others. An obscure representation of the subject's own intentions impedes the process of formulating individual life goals together with carrying out action plans and specific tasks that derive from these goals. Being unaware (or being in denial) of the fact that obstacles may arise while putting one's intentions into practice, together with a poor repertory of the specific ways to overcome these obstacles, not only reduces the chance to actually overcome them, but also affect the individual's self-image, self-esteem, sense of agency and even "life philosophy" in general (i.e. bad luck in life).

Researchers also emphasise (Trzebiński, Drogosz, 2005; Drogosz, Dziuba, Prażmowska, 2006) the importance of style in self-narratives and point out that defensive or reactive narratives that aim at the passive preservation of the subject constrain the subject. By contrast, "offensive" or "proactive" narratives that stimulate the subject's activity and maintain higher motivation levels over a long period of time (see. a "narrative of desire" in Śleszyński's phenomenological-existential approach, 1998).

The degree of narrative structuring

As frequently observed in literature, it is not their separate components that constitute the beneficial nature of self-narratives, but the way these components are structured into a coherent whole. Interestingly enough, this is not so much about one-time structuring of a coherent and complex narrative, but rather about remaining in the process of constructing a better, more coherent and better structured story. Such a story should meet specific formal and structural conditions and be based on a specific pattern of the frequency of key word categories. A seminal paper in this respect, "Do good stories produce good health?," (Ramirez-Esparza, Pennebaker, 2006, 214–215) formulates it thus:

> Constructing a story is more powerful than having a story (…), those people who increase in the use of important emotion and cognitive categories from the first to the last day of writing are the ones who benefit. Ironically, whose, who use a high rate of these words on the first day of writing are unlikely to show health improvements. Taken together, those findings suggest that those who are changing in the ways they are thinking about their emotional upheavals are the ones most likely to benefit.

On a different level of analysis, this corresponds with the directive to construct personal identities so that their boundaries could be subsequently transgressed and the previously meaningful narrative patterns could be revised and transformed in such a way that could do justice to individual experience.

Formal aspects of narrative structuring

Continuity and mutual relations within the accepted temporal axis, causal relations, clear beginning, development of the action and ending ("good stories anticipate an ending," Charme, 1984; Ślazyk, Chmielewska-Łuczak, 2008) are considered formal aspects of healthy narrative structuring. However, the previously mentioned degree to which the main character is articulated in the narrative shapes its coherence and is regarded as one of the leading factors in this respect. It is assumed (Bruner, 1990) that a better articulation of the character in the story translates into a higher degree of the story's narrative quality and its coherence, especially when the character has a strong and independent internal perspective that allows individuals to confront the rules governing the world or create them from the very beginning (Stemplewska-Żakowicz, Zalewski, 2010). At the same time, from the perspective of resilience, the ability to complete stories from the past becomes an important issue, which in turn allows individuals to make the most of the biographical potential deposited in other temporal dimensions. As an important pattern of relational health, narrative coherence can be measured by means of specially designed scales such as the *Life Story Coherence Scale* (Baerger, McAdams, 1999) and *Narrative Coherence Rating Scale* Lysaker et al., 2002).

The selected criteria that have been adopted by researchers to assess narrative coherence transcend the classic definition of the concept, thus indicating such cognitive competences of individual narrators as being able to notice contradictions within their own stories or being able to independently explain inconsistencies in their meanings, without discarding those elements of experience that fail to fit in with the story in its entirety (Androutspoulou et al., 2004). These researchers, as they particularly emphasise the necessity to use relational thought processes when narrating life experiences, point out that the audience of the narrative should also be taken into account so that narrators could realise what their listeners' needs are and how to meet them. This in turn is be possible if narrators fail to understand their own feelings and emotions.

The frequency of key word categories

References to linguistic indicators, especially to the frequency of key word categories, whose occurrence, as noticed by researchers, is correlated with the structuring of the text, is yet another strategy to identify the basic indicators of *beneficial life stories* (Pennebaker et al., 1997). By contrast to the previously mentioned data concerning the impact of the narrative structuring of experience, some researchers (Ramirez-Esparza, Pennebaker, 2006, p. 215) claim that it is the selection and frequency of a given word category that constitutes the beneficial nature of self-narratives:

> However, what predicts health improvement, is not necessarily being able to write a coherent story – with a clear beginning, middle, and – but, what helps individuals is just to tell a story, in other words to express thoughts and feelings. In addition, we can define a good narrative by looking at linguistic markers that result in healthy outcomes. In short, we conclude that good narratives are not coherent, but good narratives are those whose linguistic markers predict health and well-being.

A computer assisted analysis of key word frequency in *beneficial life stories* (Ramirez-Esparza, Pennebaker, *ibid.*) demonstrates that these words belong to the following categories: negative and positive emotion words, cognitive markers (e.g., casual words), standard function word categories (1st, 2nd, and 3rd person pronouns, articles, prepositions) and various content categories (e.g. religion, death, occupation). Language dimensions linked to improved health are high levels of positive emotions combined with moderate levels of negative ones and the use of certain cognitive words, especially those connected with causality (e.g., *because* and *reason*) and insight (e.g., *understand* and *realise*). One of the most important findings was offered by the description of pronoun usage patterns: when people use the word "I", they are briefly paying attention to themselves (and, in "edge version" they use to gain higher rates in depression scales at the same time). When using other pronouns, they are more interconnected with others (and lower on depression scales). The essence of the healing process lies in perspective switching in pronouns usage rather than in their stable, unmovable level. All those relations leads to the specific pattern of making the experience the personally meaningful and socially healthy (Kaufman, Sexton, 2006; Pennebaker, Graybeal, 2001).

Differentiation and flexibility

Both the differentiation and flexibility of self-narratives constitute their adaptive complexity that protects individuals from two threats: narrative chaos or ossification. ("Complexity implies two processes: differentiation and integration," Csikszentmihalyi, 1996, 413). Stories that are told in a differentiated manner gain both in logic and flexibility (Siegel, 2011, p. 99). This effect can be achieved through the process of thematising experience whereby order and hierarchy are established among the primarily disparate elements of individual experience. Csikszentmihalyi describes this resilience-promoting effect as a capacity for creating order out of chaos or a factor that transforms the effect of the trauma into a challenge which in turn restores meaning in one's life. This capacity can be found in individuals with *autotelic personality*, which in turn can be described as internally diverse and relatively independent from its environment. By discovering or creating a life theme individuals not only give meaning to their experience, but also are able to fight entropy experienced by others. The narrative dimension of this complex process can already be identified at the early stages of individual development as the recollections of adults who construct coherent life themes (when compared with individuals who find it difficult to identify such themes) contain considerably more scenes from their childhood in which they read or share stories with adults. This corresponds with the thesis propounded by Ricoeur (1992) whereby one can look at literature in its entirety as a laboratory of mental experiments that can be applied by people themselves, so that they can "(...) develop a powerful and useful existence" (Csikszentmihalyi, 1996, p. 406).

Content rules of the narrative interpretation of experience

Apart from the formal qualities of self-narrative structures that are beneficial to individual health and resilience, one should also pay attention to the content rules of the narrative interpretation of experience. It is not only the way in which the story is being told, but also its content that can differentiate the functioning of their narrators. The key skill seems to be harmonising inside the one life story the important universal themes (e.g. *agency and communion*, McAdams et al., 1996). Identified and described by McAdams (2006b) so called *redemptive stories*, i.e. narratives that intensify generative themes (understood as needs to support younger generations, which actualise through specific actions) are regarded as one of the best developed examples in this respect also. Intertwined with individual life stories, the theme of "being for others" helps to foster important and culturally universal values and attach meaning to these values. In certain circumstances, stories that are structured around the themes of supporting others and leaving a recognisable trace in the world may even be used as a last resort to avoid taking stock of one's life (Oleś, 2011; Tokarska, 2013).

The subjective and existential aspect of life stories

The narrative context in the definition of mental health, with a particular emphasis on resilience in the face of difficult situations, has to be considered using the subjective and existential aspect of life stories constructed by individuals. One of the main functions of the narrative structuring of experience is to make life more coherent and meaningful and enhance the individual's sense of agency. By constructing life stories, individuals can become more sensitive to narratives (subjective positions, internal worlds) created by others and can find it easier to integrate various temporal perspectives (with a particular emphasis on future-oriented narratives (Seligman et al., 2013). All this means that they form an incredibly valuable source in the process of supporting personal development (Tokarska, 2006, 2009). The ability to cope with significant and unavoidable circumstances inherent in human existence without falling victim to permanent depersonalisation (Adamiec, 1988; Viorst, 1986) and the capacity for conscious and responsible co-authoring of one's own biography is referred to in literature as "existential adaptation (Gałdowa, 1992; Kenyon, 2000; LaGrand, 1988). In the context of the main topic of this article, existential adaptation may be defined as the ability to cope with life on a deeper level whereby, instead of denying problems, individuals reflect on them in a broader perspective of their lives and their multi-layered structures (Tokarska, 2010b). The narrative mode of processing experience, which supports such a type of experiencing the world, may allow individuals to experience life in its entirety, on the condition that it produces a "good" and "beneficial" narrative. Thus understood, health is not identical with mental well-being and is closer to concepts such as growth, maturing or attaining wisdom. Health is thus related to such psychological areas of reflection as a *sense of meaning of life* (Frankl, 1998; Lucas, 1998), *sense of coherence* (Antonovsky, 1987) or *biographical competence* (Pietrasiński, 1993; Tokarska, 2011a).

The process in which individuals identify and recount their existential difficulties in a narrative form is closely related, both in theory and in practice, to *existential counselling* (Popielski, 1987; Piorunek, 2011). In such a context, it appears that the narrative approach to autobiographic material provides valuable tools to support the "process of personal growth defined in terms of the change of the perspective in which individuals perceive themselves and the world (...)" (Straś-Romanowska, 2005a, p. 104). At the same time, when individuals lose contact with their narrative identity or when something affects the role their narratives play in the process of constituting their identities, they may experience an increased sense of suffering, which, on the one hand, may upset the very act of narration and, on the other, may activete it. Simultaneously, difficult themes in human existence, if they are intentionally developed and rendered in suitable proportions within a life story, cease to be experienced as an obstacle or difficulty and, thus, become an inherent and meaningful part of the individual's life.

The narrative promotion of mental health and resilience

Since the process of achieving subsequent stages of development and narrative complexity, which is in itself beneficial to mental health and resilience, does not always take place automatically and may require external assistance (Stemplewska-Żakowicz, Zalewski, 2010), the concept of the *narrative promotion of mental health and resilience* (Tokarska, 2002, 2004, 2011c) emerges as an interesting area to develop in a therapeutic practice. Narrative therapists should thus keep in mind the concept of the development of narrative needs and tasks inherent in the entire human life cycle (Tokarska, 2010a) and be aware of various levels in the development of self-narratives as well as leading preventive resilience factors, both of which have been identified in the empirical studies mentioned above.

The ability to instil and maintain the habit of mature self-reflection on the meaning of life and one's own biography should be taken as a basis (not strictly narrative) for such a practice. This opens up a chance for its recipients to transcend the automatic and unconscious understanding of events, not only in special situations (e.g. critical situations) but also in everyday life. Such a type of self-reflection not only benefits the healthy functioning of individuals, but also their personal development:

> (…) individuals that leave a margin for unexpected and random events and are more willing to investigate their meaning and to find out what to do with them develop easier than those who want to remain autonomous and have full control over their lives and who (perhaps) treat threats as distractors and not developmental challenges (Oleś, 2011, p. 226).

In the context of this article, an important set of tools to support the personal development of individuals may be provided by creating the early emotional atmosphere in children's lives; maintaining the multi-layered and diverse internal content at subsequent stages of their development; and instilling the preference for the proactive narrative style, all of which are seemingly unrelated to the narrative understanding of mental health. The narrative mental health of the recipients of therapy may improve if they are confronted with coherent (literary and cinematic) narrative patterns that present a repertory of the possible intentions of the characters, together with the plans to put them into practice. (Tokarska, 2008a). Recipients may develop a complete self-narrative pattern if they are presented with stories that contain a clear description of the possible twists and turns in the plot as well as circumstances, opportunities and concrete tools used by the characters to cope with difficult life situations. It is also important to undertake activities that help recipients to put these patterns into practice; support them in the process of establishing a link between "raw" experience and its narrative symbolisation; and harmonise verbalised narrative with "narrative as action" (Tokarska, 2011b). From the narrative point of view, various exercises that develop „narrative flexibility" (Tokarska, 2008b) by using a variety of literary genres and metaphors to construct a story or reinterpreting those life stories that have become obsolete to their narrators (Tokarska, 2005a, 2007) are essential for the improvement of individual resilience levels. If the character, who is also the narrator, is clearly articulated in the story, it is easier to bring out their subjective qualities and they also find it easier to transform these qualities into intentional actions and relationships with others, which in turn benefits their sense of self-agency and makes them feels as co-authors of their life stories. It is worth taking such intentional narrative action at every stage of human development: from working with parents of unborn babies to creating favourable conditions for senior individuals to help them find meaning in their lives.

References

Adamiec, M. (1988). *Doświadczenie przemiany jako kategoria psychologiczna.* Katowice: Wydawnictwo Uniwersytetu Śląskiego.

Androutsopoulou, A., Thanopoulou, K., Economou, E., Bafiti, T. (2004). Forming criteria for assessing the coherence of clients' life stories: a narrative study. *Journal of Family Therapy*, 26 (4), 384–406.

Antonovsky, A. (1987). *Unraveling the Mystery of Health.* San Francisco: Jossey-Bass. [Polish version: Antonovsky, A. (1995). *Rozwikłanie tajemnicy zdrowia,* Warszawa: Fundacja IPN].

Baerger, D., McAdams, D. (1999). Life story coherence, its reliability to psychological well-being. *Narrative Inquiry*, (9), 1, 69–96.

Baikie, K., Wilhelm, K. (2005). Emotional and physical health benefits of expressive writing. *Advances of Psychiatric Treatment*, 11, 338–346.

Błaszczak, W. (2002). *Poczucie zmiany osobowości po doświadczeniu realnego zagrożenia życia,* nieopublikowana praca doktorska.

Botella, L., Herrero, O. (2000). A Relational Constructivist Approach to Narrative Therapy. *European Journal of Psychotherpy, Counselling and Health*, (3), 3, 407–418.

Bruner, J. (1986). *Actual Minds, Possible Worlds.* Cambridge: Harvard University Press.

76

Bruner, J. (1990). Życie jako narracja, *Kwartalnik Pedagogiczny*, 4, 3–17.

Campbell, R., Pennebaker, J. (2003). The secret life of pronouns: Flexibility in writing style and physical health. *Psychological Science*, 14, 60–65.

Carr, A. (1998). Michael White's Narrative Therapy. *Contemporary Family Therapy*, 20, 4, 485–503.

Charme, S. (1984). *Meaning and Myth in the Study of Lives: A Sartrean Perspective.* Philadelphia: University of Pennsylvania Press.

Chrzczonowicz, A. (2011). Narracja w psychiatrii – teoria, zastosowanie, związki ze zdrowiem psychicznym. *Postępy Psychiatrii i Neurologii*, 20, 4, 283–289.

Cozolino, L. (2002). *The Neuroscience of Psychotherapy: Building and Rebuilding the Human Brain.* W.W. Norton. [Polish version: Cozolino. New York (2004). *Neuronauka w psychoterapii. Budowa i przebudowa ludzkiego umysłu.* Poznań: Zysk i S-ka Wydawnictwo].

Csikszentmihalyi, M. (1992). *Flow: the Psychology of Happiness.* London: Rider. [Polish version: Csikszentmihalyi, M. (1996). *Przepływ. Psychologia optymalnego doświadczenia.* Warszawa: Wydawnictwo Studio Emka].

Denett, D. (1992). The Self as a center of narrative gravity. [In:] F. Kessel, P. Cole, D. Johnson (Eds.). *Self and Consciousness: Multiple Perspectives.* Hillsdale: Erlbaum.

Denham, A. (2008). Rethinking Historical Trauma: Narratives of Resilience. *Transcultural Psychiatry*, 45 (3), 391–414.

Dimaggio, G., Salvatore, G., Azzara, C., Catania, D., Semenari, A., Hermans, H. (2003). Dialogical relationships in impoverished narratives: From theory to clinical practice. *Psychology and Psychotherapy: Theory, Research and Practice*, 76, 385–409.

Dimaggio, G., Semenari, A. (2001). Psychopathological narrative forms. *Journal of Constructivist Psychology*, 14, 1–23.

Drogosz, M., Dziuba, M., Prażmowska, M. (2006). Styl autonarracji a wybrane aspekty funkcjonowania członków różnych grup społecznych. *Psychologia Jakości Życia*, 5, 213–236.

Dryll, E. (2010). Wielkie i małe narracje w życiu człowieka. [In:] M. Straś-Romanowska, B. Bartosz, M. Żurko (Eds.). *Badania narracyjne w psychologii.* Warszawa: Eneteia, Wydawnictwo Psychologii i Kultury, 163–182.

Frankl, V. (1998). *Homo Patiens.* Warszawa: Instytut Wydawniczy Pax.

Gałdowa, A. (1992). *Powszechność i wyjątek. Rozwój osobowości człowieka dorosłego.* Kraków: Wydawnictwo Uniwersytetu Jagiellońskiego.

Giddens, A. (1991). *Modernity and Self-identity. Self and Society in the Modern Age.* Stanford: Stanford University Press.

Greenberg, I., Angus, L. (2004). *The Contribution of Emotion Processes to Narrative Change in Psychotherapy. Practice, Theory, Research.* London–New Delhi: Sage Publications.

Grzegorek, A. (2005). Jak mówienie zmienia myślenie? [In:] A. Niedźwieńska (Ed.). *Zmiana osobowości. Wybrane zagadnienia.* Kraków: Wydawnictwo Uniwersytetu Jagiellońskiego, 121–129.

Hauser, S., Allen, J., Golden, E. (2006). *Out the Woods: Tales of Teen Resilience.* Cambridge: Harvard University Press.

Hauser, S., Allen, J. (2007). Overcoming Adversity in Adolescence: Narratives of Resilience, *Psychoanalytic Inquiry*, 26 (4), 549–576.

Hermans, H., Kempen, H. (1993). *The Dialogical Self: Meaning as Movement.* San Diego: Academic Press.

Hermans, H., Hermans-Jansen, E. (1995). *Self-narratives: The Construction of Meaning in Psychotherapy.* New York: Guilford Press. [Polish version: Hermans, H., Hermans-Jansen, E. (2000). *Autonarracje. Tworzenie znaczeń w psychoterapii.* Warszawa: Pracownia Testów Psychologicznych Polskiego Towarzystwa Psychologicznego].

Hermans, H. (1996). Voicing the self: From information processing to dialogical interchange. *Psychological Bulletin,* 119, 31–50.

Hermans, H. (1999). Self-Narrative as Meaning Construction: The Dynamics ol Self-lnvestigation, *Journal of Clinical Psychology,* 55 (10), 1193–1211.

Janusz, B., Gdowska, K., de Barbaro, B. (Eds.) (2008). *Narracja. Teoria i praktyka.* Kraków: Wydawnictwo Uniwersytetu Jagielońskiego.

Juczyński, Z. (2012). *Coping with pain and suffering – towards mobilization of personal resources for health.* [In:] D. Kubacka-Jasiecka, M. Kuleta (Eds.). *Reflections on Psychological Mechanisms of Trauma and Posttraumatic Development.* Kraków: Wydawnictwo Kontekst, 163–177.

Kaufman, J., Sexton, J. (2006). Why doesn't Writing Cure Help Poets? *Review of General Psychology,* 10 (3), 268–282.

Keen, S. (1986). *Faces of the Enemy: Reflections of the Hostile Imagination.* San Francisco: Harper Row.

Kenyon, G. (2000). *Philosophical foundations of existential meaning.* [In:] G. Reker, K. Chamberlain (Eds.). *Exploring Existential Meaning: Optimizing Human Development Across the Life Span.* Thousand Oaks CA: Sage, 7–22.

Kleinman, A. (1988). *The Illness Narratives. Suffering, Healing, the Human Condition.* New York: Basic Books.

Kozłowska-Piwowarczyk, I. (2008). *Narracje biofilne – wspierające rozwój, a narracje nekrofilne – hamujące rozwój.* [In:] B. Janusz, K. Gdowska, B. de Barbaro (Eds.). *Narracja. Teoria i praktyka.* Kraków: Wydawnictwo Uniwersytetu Jagiellońskiego, 507–521.

Kubacka-Jasiecka, D., Kuleta, M. (Eds.) (2012). *Reflections on Psychological Mechanisms of Trauma and Posttraumatic Development.* Kraków: Wydawnictwo Kontekst.

LaGrand, L. (1988). *Changing Patterns of Human Existence: Assumptions, Beliefs, and Coping with the Stress of Change.* Springfield, Illinois: C.C. Thomas Publishing.

Lepore, S., Smyth, J. (2002). *The Writing Cure: How Expressive Writing Promotes Health and Emotional Well-Being.* Washington: American Psychological Association.

Lucas, E. (1998). *The meaning of life and the goals in life for chronically ill people.* [In:] P. Wong, P. Fry (Eds.). *The Human Quest for Meaning.* Mahwah, NJ: Lawrence Erlbaum Associates, 307–316.

Lysaker, P., Lysaker, J. (2001). Schizophrenia and the collapse of the dialogical self: Recovery, narrative and psychotherapy. Psychotherapy, 38, 3, 252–261.

Lysaker, P., Clements, C., Plascak-Hallberg, C., Knipscheer, S., Wright, D. (2002). Insight and personal narratives of illness in schizophrenia, *Psychiatry,* 65, 197–206.

Lysaker, P., Wicket, A., Wilke, N., Lysaker, J. (2003a), Narrative incoherence in schizophrenia. The absent agent-protagonist and the collapse of internal dialogue. *American Journal of Psychotherapy,* 57, 153–166.

Lysaker, P., Lancaster, R., Lysaker, J. (2003b), Narrative transformation as an outcome in the psychotherapy of schizophrenia, *Psychology and Psychotherapy: Theory, Research and Practice,* 76, 285–299.

Lysaker, P., Lysaker, J. (2006). A typology of narrative impoverishment in schizopphrenia: Implications for understanding the process of establishing and sustaining dialogue in individual psychotherapy. *Counselling Psychology Quartely*, 19, 57–68.

Lyubomirsky, S., Sousa, L., Dickerhoof, R. (2006). The Cost and Benefits of Writing, Talking and Thinking About Life's Triumphs and Defeats. *Journal of Personality and Social Psychology*, 90 (4), 692–708.

Łoś, Z. (2010). *Rozwój psychiczny człowieka w ciągu całego życia.* Wrocław: Wydawnictwo Uniwersytetu Wrocławskiego.

Mansfield, C., McLean, K., Lilgendahl, J. (2010). Narrating traumas and transgressions. Links between narrative processing, wisdom and well-being. *Narrative Inquiry*, 20 (2), 246–273.

McAdams, D. (2006b), *Redemptive Self: Stories Americans Live By.* Oxford, New York: Oxford University Press.

McAdams, D., Hoffman, B., Mansfield, E., Day, R. (1996). Themes of agency and communion in significant autobiographical scenes. *Journal of Personality*, 64, 339–378.

Morgan, A. (2000). *What is narrative therapy. An easy-to-read introduction.* Australia: Dulwich Centre Publications. [Polish version: Morgan, A. (2011). *Terapia narracyjna. Wprowadzenie.* Warszawa: Wydawnictwo Paradygmat].

Neckar, J. (2000). Narracyjne ujęcie „ja" na tle innych sposobów jego ujmowania. [In:] A. Gałdowa (Ed.). *Tożsamość człowieka.* Kraków: Wydawnictwo Uniwersytetu Jagiellońskiego, 139–148.

Nochi, M. (1998). „Loss of Self" in the narratives of people with traumatic brain injuries: a qualitative analysis. *Social Science Medicine*, 46, 869–878.

Ochs, E., Capps, L. (1996). Narrating the Self. *Annual Review of Anthropology*, 25, 19–43.

Oleś, P. (2011). *Psychologia człowieka dorosłego. Ciągłość – zmiana – integracja.* Warszawa: Wydawnictwo Naukowe PWN.

Pennebaker, J. (1997). *Openig Up: The Healing Power of Expressing Emotions.* New York: Guilford. [Polish version: Pennebaker, J. (2001). *Otwórz się. Uzdrawiająca siła wyrażania emocji.* Poznań: Media Rodzina].

Pennebaker, J., Mayne, T., Francis, M. (1997). Linguistic predictors of adaptive bereavement, *Journal of Personality and Social Psychology,* 72, 863–871.

Pennebaker, J., Seagal, D. (1999). Forming a Story: The Health Benefits of Narrative. *Journal of Clinical Psychology*, 55 (10), 1243–1254.

Pennebaker, J., Graybeal, A. (2001). Patterns of natural language use. Disclosure, personality, and social integration. *Current Directions*, 10, 90–93.

Pennebaker, J., Chung, C. (2007). *Expressive writing, emotional upheavals and health.* [In:] H. Friedman, R. Silver (Eds.). *Handbook of Health Psychology.* New York: Oxford University Press.

Pietrasiński, Z. (1993). *Syntezy wiedzy autobiograficznej podporządkowane roli autokreacyjnej jednostki.* [In:] J. Leoński, T. Rzepa (Eds.). *O biografii i metodzie biograficznej.* Poznań: Wydawnictwo Nakom, 53–71.

Piorunek, M. (Ed.) (2011). *Poradnictwo. Kolejne przybliżenia.* Toruń: Wydawnictwo Adam Marszałek.

Popielski, K. (1987). *Człowiek – pytanie otwarte.* Lublin: Wydawnictwo Katolickiego Uniwersytetu Lubelskiego.

Ramirez-Esparza, N., Pennebaker, J. (2006). Do good stories produce good health? Exploring words, language and culture. *Narrative Inquiry*, 16, 211–219.

Real, T. (2009). *Nie chcę o tym mówić. Studium męskiej depresji.* Warszawa: Wydawnictwo Czarna Owca.

Richert, A. (2002). The Self in Narrative Therapy: Thoughts from Humanistic/Existential Perspective. *Journal of Psychotherapy Integration*, 12, 1, 77–104.

Richert, A. (2003). Living Stories, Telling Stories, Changing Stories: Experiential Use of the Relationship in Narrative Therapy. *Journal of Psychotherapy Integration*, 13, 2, 210.

Ricoeur, P. (1992). *Filozofia osoby.* Warszawa: PAT.

Salvatore, G., Dimaggio, G., Semenari, A. (2004). A model of narrative development: Implications for understanding psychopathology and guiding therapy. *Psychology and Psychotherapy: Theory, Research, Practice*, 77, 231–254.

Sarbin Th. (Ed.) (1986). *Narrative Psychology: the Storied Nature of Human Conduct.* New York: Preager.

Seligman, M., Railton, P., Baumaister, R., Sripada Ch. (2013). Navigation Into the Future or Driven by the Past. *Perspectives on Psychological Science*, 8, (2), 119–141.

Shostrom, E. (1972). *Freedom to Be: Experiencing and Expressing Your Total Being.* New York: Bantam Books Inc.

Siegel, D. (2010). *Mindsight. The New Science of Personal Transformation.* New York: Random House, Bantam Books. [Polish version: Siegel, D. (2011). *Psychowzroczność. Przekształć własny umysł zgodnie z regułami nowej wiedzy o empatii.* Poznań: Wydawnictwo Media Rodzina].

Soroko, E. (2008). *Zmiana w terapiach narracyjnych.* [In:] J. Słapińska (Ed.). *Pojęcie zmiany w teorii i praktyce psychologicznej.* Poznań: Wydawnictwo Naukowe UAM, 91–120.

Soroko, E. (2012). *Beneficial effects of writing and narration in the context of a traumatic experience.* [In:] D. Kubacka-Jasiecka, M. Kuleta (Eds.). *Reflections on Psychological Mechanisms of Trauma and Posttraumatic Development.* Kraków: Wydawnictwo Kontekst, 215–241.

Stemplewska-Żakowicz, K. (2001). *Umysł dyskursywny. Propozycje teoretyczne podejścia dyskursywnego w psychologii.* [In:] I. Kurcz, J. Bobryk, (red.). *Psychologiczne studia nad językiem i dyskursem.* Warszawa: Wydawnictwo Instytutu Psychologii PAN i SWPS.

Stemplewska-Żakowicz, K. (2002). *„Wewnętrzna demokracja" jako dialogowy wzorzec zdrowia psychicznego.* [In:] J. Trzebiński (Ed.). *Narracja jako sposób rozumienia świata.* Gdańsk: Gdańskie Wydawnictwo Psychologiczne, 109–112.

Stemplewska-Żakowicz, K. (2004). *O rzeczach widywanych na obrazkach i opowiadanych o nich historiach. TAT jako metoda badawcza i diagnostyczna.* Warszawa: Wydawnictwo Akacemica SWPS.

Stemplewska-Żakowicz, K., Zalewski, B. (2010). *Czym jest dobra narracja? Struktura narracji z perspektywy badaczy i klinicystów.* [In:] M. Straś-Romanowska, B. Bartosz, M. Żurko (Eds.). *Badania narracyjne w* psychologii. Warszawa: Eneteia, Wydawnictwo Psychologii i Kultury, 17–51.

Stiles, W., Honos-Webb, L., Lani, J. (1999). Some functions of narrative in the assimilation of problematic experiences. *Journal of Clinical Psychology*, 55 (10), 1213–1226.

Straś-Romanowska, M. (2005a). *Zmiana pozycji narracyjnej podmiotu jako przejaw jego rozwoju. Analiza biograficzna wybranych postaci literackich.* [In:] E. Chmielnicka-Kuter, M. Puchalska-Wasyl, P. Oleś (Eds.). *Polifonia osobowości. Aktualne problemy psychologii narracji.* Lublin: Wydawnictwo Katolickiego Uniwersytetu Lubelskiego, 89–108.

Straś-Romanowska, M. (2005b), Jakość życia w świetle założeń psychologii zorientowanej na osobę, *Kolokwia Psychologiczne*, 13, 263–274.

Ślazyk, M., Chmielewska-Łuczak, D. (2008). *Każda historia ma swój koniec.* [In:] B. Janusz, K. Gdowska, B. de Barbaro (Eds.). *Narracja. Teoria i praktyka.* Kraków: Wydawnictwo Uniwersytetu Jagiellońskiego, 305–312.

Śleszyński, D. (1998). *Wędrówka doświadczenia. Podejście fenomenologiczne i egzystencjalne.* Bydgoszcz: Wydawnictwo Trans Humana.

Tekin, S. (2011). Self-Concept Through the Diagnostic Looking Glass: Narratives and Mental Disorder. *Philosophical Psychology*, 24 (3), 357–380.

Tokarska, U. (1994). Konstytuowanie się podmiotu przez narrację. *Zeszyty Naukowe Uniwersytetu Jagiellońskiego, Prace Psychologiczne*, 11, 59–69.

Tokarska, U. (1995, 1999). *W poszukiwaniu jedności i celu. Wybrane techniki narracyjne.* [In:] A. Gałdowa (Ed.). *Wybrane zagadnienia z psychologii osobowości.* Kraków: Wydawnictwo Uniwersytetu Jagiellońskiego, 169–204.

Tokarska, U. (2000a). *Narracja autobiograficzna w psychologicznym poznaniu i terapii. Studium teoretyczne*, nieopublikowana praca doktorska. Wrocław: Uniwersytet Wrocławski.

Tokarska, U. (2000b). *Terapia narracyjna. Założenia teoretyczne, metody pracy, obszary zastosowań.* [In:] M. Straś-Romanowska (Ed.). *Metody jakościowe w psychologii współczesnej.* Wrocław: Wydawnictwo Uniwersytetu Wrocławskiego, 185–193.

Tokarska, U. (2002). *Narracja autobiograficzna w terapii i promocji zdrowia.* [In:] J. Trzebiński (Ed.). *Narracja jako sposób rozumienia świata.* Gdańsk: Gdańskie Wydawnictwo Psychologiczne, 221–261.

Tokarska, U. (2004). *Narracja autobiograficzna we wspomaganiu rozwoju człowieka.* [In:] A. Cierpka, E. Dryll (Eds.). *Narracja. Koncepcje i badania psychologiczne.* Warszawa: Wydawnictwo Instytutu Psychologii PAN, 285–302.

Tokarska, U. (2005a). *Narracja autobiograficzna jako „opowieść drogi" w ujęciu, C. Pearson.* [In:] E. Chmielnicka-Kuter, M. Puchalska-Wasyl (Eds.). *Polifonia osobowości. Aktualne problemy psychologii narracji.* Lublin: Wydawnictwo Katolickiego Uniwersytetu Lubelskiego, 125–140.

Tokarska, U. (2006). Narracyjne strategie wspomagania rozwoju osobowego, *Psychologia Rozwojowa*, 1, 55–68.

Tokarska, U. (2007). *Archetypowe scenariusze życia a rozwój człowieka dorosłego.* [In:] K. Węgłowska-Rzepa, D. Fredericksen (Eds.). *Między świadomością a nieświadomością. Współczesność w perspektywie psychologii głębi.* Warszawa: Eneteia, Wydawnictwo Psychologii i Kultury, 277–293.

Tokarska, U. (2008a). *Wybrane strategie wykorzystania tekstów literackich w narracyjnych oddziaływaniach profilaktycznych.* [In:] B. Janusz, K. Gdowska, B. de Barbaro (Eds.). *Narracja. Teoria i praktyka.* Kraków: Wydawnictwo Uniwersytetu Jagiellońskiego, 471–499.

Tokarska, U. (2008b). *Reaching narrative unity inside the inner plurality in the dialogical context.* [In:] M. Pourkos (Ed.). *Perspectives and Limits of Dialogism in Mikhail*

Bakhtin: Applications in Psychology, Art, Education and Culture. Crete: University of Crete, 141–154.

Tokarska, U. (2009). *Wątki egzystencjalne w psychologii narracyjnej.* [In:] H. Wrona-Polańska, E. Czerniawska, L. Wrona (Eds.). *Szkice o ludzkim poznawaniu i odczuwaniu.* Kraków: Wydawnictwo Naukowe Uniwersytetu Pedagogicznego, 103–116.

Tokarska, U. (2010a). *„Stawać się Panem Własnego Oblicza". O możliwościach intencjonalnych oddziaływań narracyjnych w biegu życia ludzkiego.* [In:] M. Straś-Romanowska, B. Bartosz, M. Żurko (Eds.). *Psychologia małych i wielkich narracji.* Warszawa: Eneteia, Wydawnictwo Psychologii i Kultury, 293–314.

Tokarska, U. (2010b). *Narracyjna GRA (auto)BIOGRAFICZNA <W osiemdziesiąt historii do-o-KOŁA ŻYCIA> jako autorska metoda profilaktyki problemów egzystencjalnych współczesnego człowieka.* [In:] M. Śniarowska-Tlatlik (Ed.). *Psychologia bliżej bycia. Inspiracje egzystencjalne.* Kraków: AT Group, 133–142.

Tokarska (2011a). *Kształcenie kompetencji biograficznej jako forma profilaktyki problemów egzystencjalnych współczesnego człowieka.* [In:] M. Piorunek (Ed.). *Poradnictwo. Kolejne przybliżenia.* Toruń: Wydawnictwo Adam Marszałek, 57–81.

Tokarska, U. (2011b). *Tożsamość narracyjna w dobie płynnej nowoczesności – nowe wyzwania dla psychologii narracyjnej.* [In:] E. Litak, R. Furman, H. Brożek (Eds.). *Pejzaże tożsamości. Teoria i empiria w perspektywie interdyscyplinarnej.* Kraków: Wydawnictwo Uniwersytetu Jagiellońskiego, 37–50.

Tokarska, U. (2011c). *Narracyjna GRA (auto)BIOGRAFICZNA <W osiemdziesiąt historii do-o-KOŁA ŻYCIA> jako autorska forma wspomagania rozwoju człowieka dorosłego.* [In:] E. Dryll, A. Cierpka (Eds.). *Psychologia narracyjna. Tożsamość, dialogowość, pogranicza.* Warszawa: Eneteia, Wydawnictwo Psychologii i Kultury, 219–239.

Tokarska, U. (2013). O porzebie bycia potrzebnym. Miejsce generatywności w bilansie życiowym współczesnego człowieka. Toruń: Wydawnictwo Adam Marszałek.

Trzebiński, J. (2002). (Ed.). *Narracja jako sposób rozumienia świata.* Gdańsk: Gdańskie Wydawnictwo Psychologiczne.

Trzebiński, J. (2005). Narracyjny kontekst myślenia i działania. [In:] E. Chmielnicka-Kuter, M. Puchalska-Wasyl (Eds.). *Polifonia osobowości. Aktualne problemy psychologii narracji.* Lublin: Wydawnictwo Katolickiego Uniwersytetu Lubelskiego, 67–87.

Trzebiński, J., Drogosz, M. (2005). *Historie, które kształtują nasze życie: O konsekwencjach proaktywnych i defensywnych autonarracji.* [In:] M. Drogosz (Ed.). *Jak Polacy wygrywają, jak Polacy przegrywają.* Gdańsk: Gdańskie Wydawnictwo Psychologiczne, 149–165.

Ungar, M. (Ed.) (2012). *The Social Ecology of Resilience.* New York, London: Springer.

Viorst, J. (1986). *Necessary Losses. The Loves, Illusions, Dependencies and Impossible Expectations That All of Us Have to Give Up In Order to Grow.* US: The Free Publisher. [Polish version: Viorst, J. (1996). *To, co musimy utracić – czyli miłość, złudzenia, zależności i niemożliwe do spełnienia oczekiwania, których każdy z nas musi się wyrzec, by móc wzrastać.* Poznań: Zysk i S-ka Wydawnictwo].

White, M., Epston, D. (Eds.) (1990). *Narrative Means to Therapeutic Ends.* New York, London: W.W. Norton, CO.

White Ch., Denborough, D. (Eds.) (1999). *Introducing Narrative Therapy. A Collection of Practice-based Writings.* Adelaide: Dulwich Centre Publications.

II. RESILIENCE IN DEVELOPMENT

Iwona Sikorska
Jagiellonian University
The Institute of Applied Psychology

THEORETICAL MODELS OF RESILIENCE AND RESILIENCE MEASUREMENT TOOLS IN CHILDREN AND YOUNG PEOPLE

Abstract

The definitional problems related to the concept of resilience show that it may be understood in a variety of ways (Masten, 2001; Richardson, 2002; Masten, Obradović, 2006; Kolar, 2011). Primarily, it is described as successful adaptation and successful development despite external risks. Researchers argue that individuals may be referred to as resilient only if they faced real external threats to their development (e.g. mental illness in the family, their low social and economic standing, violence) and yet were able to cope and develop properly (Luthar, 1999; Masten, 2001; Borucka, Ostaszewski, 2008; Kolar, 2011). The phenomenon of resilience may also be defined as a dynamic process whereby an interaction between risk and protection factors occurs, both on an individual and social level. In this case the researchers focus on mechanisms that modify risk factors. Yet another approach aims to define a set of personal traits that may be referred to as ego-resiliency (Block, 1980; Constantine et al., 1999). Every approach to the phenomenon of resilience offers its own theoretical models and measurement tools.

This paper focuses on resilience in developmental age. It aims to present selected resilience measurement scales and component skills in children and young people. The selected measurement tools are following: Kidscreen (Polish adaptation: Mazur, Małkowska-Szkutnik, Dzielska, Tabak, 2008), The Healthy Kids Survey (HKS, 1999), DECA (LeBuffe, Naglieri, 1998), DESSA (LeBuffe, Naglieri, Shapiro, 2006), and Resilience Scale SPP 18 (Ogińska-Bulik, Juczyński, 2011).

Key words: developmental age, resilience, measurement

The current state of knowledge in the field

"Resilience is a broad conceptual umbrella, covering many concepts related to positive patterns of adaptation in the context of adversity. The conceptual family of resilience encompasses a class of phenomena where the adaptation of a system has been threatened by experiences of disrupting or destroying the successful operations of the system" (Masten, Obradović, 2006, p. 14).

Definitional considerations

An important basis for a better understanding of individual resilience resources has been provided by longitudinal studies on children growing up in difficult circumstances and on factors that reduce risk in the process of children's development. These studies include: the longitudinal study carried out on the Hawaiian island of Kauai, USA (Werner, 2000), the study on Children at Risk in Mannheim, Germany (Laucht et al., 2000), and the study on vulnerability in Bielefeld, Germany (Andre/Loesel, 1997, 1998 by: Wustmann, 2004). The results of these studies have reshaped our current understanding of children's capacity to overcome adversity and deal with developmental risks. Researchers have started to consider not only potential confounders, but also those factors that are conducive to good health. Thus, a change in the approach to *mental health* has occurred, shifting the perspective from pathogenic to a salutogenic one. Attention has been paid not only to resilience deficits and deficiencies, but also to resources and competencies that help overcome strains and stresses as well as obstacles. In addition to risk factors, particular attention has been paid to protective factors (Antonovsky, 1995; Werner, 2000; Tugade, Fredrikson, Feldman Barrett, 2004).

A historical perspective on the concept of resilience and its development over time allows one to notice earlier studies dealing with essentially the same phenomenon, namely a phenomenon of good health in spite of being exposed to prolonged and severe stress. Researchers tried to explain it by means of personality constructs, such as resistance or hardiness proposed by Kobasa (1979) and a sense of coherence (SOC) proposed by Antonovsky (1979) (Zwolinski, 2011).

Resilience is considered to be an important feature of personality, conducive to good health and a "key to it" and, as such, may also be regarded as a "meta-source" of special regulatory power, influencing the activation of other resources needed in the process of coping with life events (Ogińska-Bulik, Juczyński, 2011).

The analysis of the ways in which resilience has been conceptualized and operationalised in the field of human development allows one to present four major branches of research on children and adolescents.

Development in the field – theory and research

1. The first and pioneering branch of research dates back to the 1970s. It focusses on the psychopathology of children and adolescents and seeks causes of major mental disorders in children and adolescents (Garmezy, 1971; Murphy, 1974; Rutter, 1979). This branch of research draws attention to children that develop well despite their negative genetic endowment or hostile environment. First reports of this kind have shed light on children resilient to injury and with extraordinary qualities (Masten, 2001). Thus, the question have arisen about the correlates and determinants for a s u c c e s s f u l a d a p t a t i o n. The researchers have also described a number of internal assets of children and young people and protective factors conducive to coping in spite of adversity, living in difficult conditions or experiencing a trauma.

The researchers assume that an individual can be referred to as resilient if their normal development has been put at risk (e.g. because of the mental illness of their parent, low social and economic status of their family or domestic violence) and yet they have been able to cope with the situation and develop successfully.

The researchers have also found out that numerous risk factors tend to coincide in children's life. In addition to potential risks and threats, internal assets have also been highlighted and it has been established that the higher is their level, the better results children and adolescents achieve in terms of positive adaptation (Luthar, 1999; Masten, 2001; Borucka, Ostaszewski, 2008; Kolar, 2011). This branch of research also studies the criteria according to which the process of adaptation can be described as successful or satisfactory. One such criterion helps to assess the process of completing developmental tasks as it indicates whether children develop in compliance with cultural expectations typical of their age or whether they learn competencies they are expected to acquire. Yet another perspective on the criteria for successful adaptation highlights the non-occurrence of psychopathological behavior as well as low levels of distress. The outcome of successful adaptation would thus manifest itself as mental health, social competence and the ability to take action (Olsson et al., 2003, as cited [In:] Kolar, 2011).

2. The second branch of research offers a slightly different understanding of resilience, thus describing it as a dynamic p r o c e s s, whereby an interaction between risk factors and both external and internal protective factors takes place. This branch of research pays particular attention to mechanisms that may influence and modify risk factors. The analysis of its results demonstrates that resilience is contextual and prone to change, which in turn provides an argument against reducing this phenomenon to merely a repeated way in which individuals respond to risk factors (Masten, 2001; Olsson et al., 2003; Coleman, Hagell, 2007; as cited [In:] Kolar, 2011).

Research on resilience as a process treats it as an ability that develops over time as a result of interaction between an individual and their environment. The analysed aspects of this interaction include children's temperament levels and intelligence quotient, mother-child relationship, the quality of parenting and home environment, symptoms of depressive disorders in the family, socio-economic status, traumatic family events and family support (England et al., 1993, as cited [In:] Kolar, 2011). Projects carried out according to these criteria are primarily concerned with response to enduring stressors.

3. The third branch of research puts emphasis on the application of knowledge in the field of resilience. Prevention, intervention and creating a protective system are thus regarded as activities that play a particularly important role in instilling resilience in children and adolescents living in conditions detrimental to their normal development. Projects carried out by these researchers have shown that external and internal assets can make a significant contribution to the development of resilience (Liebenberg, Unger, 2009; as cited [In:] Kolar, 2011). Research according to these guidelines has been conducted in Poland, too, by Joanna Mazur from the Institute of Mother and Child and the team of researchers under guidance of Krzysztof Ostaszewski from the Institute of Psychiatry and Neurology in Warsaw.

4. Developed at the conference on Resilience in Children in 2006, the fourth branch of research stems from the other three and primarily aims to integrate all the fields of research on resilience in children through multilevel analyses as well as interdisciplinary and cross-generic approach. This approach calls for co-operation and exchange between various fields of research, including genetics, neuroscience and behavioral biology. The fourth branch of research on resilience gives hope for a better and more thorough understanding of processes and multilevel relations involved in resilience (Masten, 2006; Kolar, 2011).

Figure 1 summarizes theoretical assumptions in various resilience research.

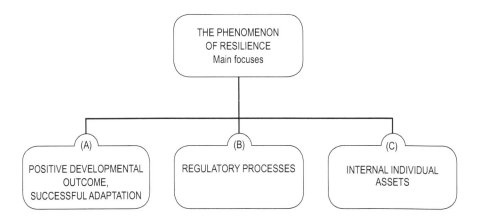

Figure 1. Theoretical models of resilience (on Masten, 2006; Kolar, 2011)

Research designs and examples of measurement tools

The respective objects of study allow one to identify two models of research on resilience in children:

The first model is a variable-focused one. The variables analyzed by this branch of research include: the socioeconomic status (SES) (McLoyd, 1998; Luthar, 1991, 2000), parenting quality (Malmberg, Flouri, 2011) parent-child relationship (McCubbin, 1993; Masten, 2001), measurable genetic polymorphism (Greenberg et al., 2007 in Kolar, 2011) and intellectual functioning (Masten, Obradović, 2006). The results for these variables have been achieved in the areas such as results at school, social and antisocial behavior, peer acceptance or psychopathological behavior (Luthar, 1991; Masten, 2001; Masten, Obradović, 2006).

The second approach is a person-focused one. At first, this branch of research provides individual case studies of children that have overcome a trauma or coped with adverse conditions (e.g. losing a parent in early childhood). Then it offers multiple case studies that allow one to identify recurring patterns in the development of children with similar life experiences (e.g. studies on adopted Romanian children living in orphanages prior to their adoption) (Masten, O'Connor, 1989; Ames, 1997). The person-focused approach adheres to the assumptions of classical longitudinal methodology, used in such studies as The Kauai Study by Werner and Smith as well as The Rochester Resilience Study by Cowen, Wyman et al. (Werner, Smith, 1992; Wyman et al., 1999).

The list of tools for measuring competency indicative of mental health in children and adolescents have been provided by Darlene Kordich Hall (2010). This list includes 38 different tools that help to measure competences connected with resilience. H a r d i n e s s level in children can be recognized by the Psychological Hardiness Scale (PHS) (Younkin, Betz, 1996) for adolescents and adults. Children's s t r e n g t h s can be in turn measured by the Strengths and Difficulties Questionnaire for children from 3 to 18 years of age (SDQ) (Goodman, 1997) or the Emotional and Behavioral Development Scale for children aged 5 to 16 (EBDS) (Riding, Rayner, Morris et al., 2002). P r o t e c t i v e f a c t o r s a n d r i s k f a c t o r s in adolescents are, for example, measured using the Rochester Evaluation of Asset Development for Youth (READY) (Klein et al., 2006).

Research on r e s i l i e n c e in children and adolescents takes advantage of tools such as observation scales, completed by parents, carers and teachers, including the DESSA, namely the Devereux Student Strengths Assessment (LeBuffe, Naglieri, Shapiro, 2006) or self-reporting methods designed for older students such as the Child, Youth Resilience Measure (CYRM)) for students aged from 12 to 23 (Ungar, Leibenberg, 2009).

Theoretical framework and measurement example

Resilience as a positive developmental outcome

„Resilience should to be seen as an acquired, gradually internalized set of attributes that enable a person to adapt to life's difficult circumstances" (Alvord, Grados, 2005, p. 244).

The first theoretical proposal is connected with variable-focused studies of resilience. Figure 3 shows some kind of main effects for an assets variable, risk-adversity variable, along with the bipolar predictor. It has been found out that not only risks and internal assets, but also bipolar predictors have also been highlighted. All these groups of factors influence results, which children and adolescents achieve in terms of positive adaptation. Desirable outcome in children includes external adaptation criteria (academic achievements) and internal adaptation criteria (psychological well-being, absence of psychopathology) (Luthar, 1999; Masten, 2001).

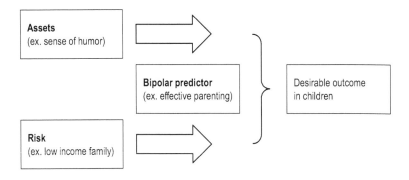

Figure 2. Resilience as outcome (on Masten, 2001)

The Kidscreen Questionnaire can be given as a measurement tool based on this theoretical framework.

The Kidscreen Project was implemented in 13 European countries including Poland, during the years 2003–2004, within the Fifth Framework Programme (research related to Health Related Quality of Life). Six questionnaires were developed for studying the health related quality of life in children and adolescents aged 8–18, including a full, intermediate and short version, each with an option for a child and for a parent or caregiver responding on behalf of the child. At the end of 2006 an international manual was published in English and 2008 in Polish (Polish adaptation by Mazur, Małkowska-Szkutnik, Dzielska and Tabak). On the basis of Polish data, the structure and psychometric properties of the Kidscreen-52 Questionnaire was described (child version), and a comparison was made between the answers to the questions put in the full scale by children and parents. The quality of life is measured in a a full (52 items), intermediate (27 items) and short (10 items) version in 10 following fields.

Table 1. Kidscreen Questionnaire (after Mazur, Małkowska-Szkutnik, Dzielska and Tabak, 2008)

Questionnaire instruction: *Thinking about last week answer the questions:*

Individual development	Context of development
1. Physical health *Were you full of energy?*	6. Parent-child relation *Did your parents understand you?*
2. Mental health *Did you have a good time?*	7. Socio-economic status *Did you have enough money for your needs and pleasures?*
3. Emotional wellbeing *Did you feel lonely?*	8. Peers and social support *Did you spend time with your friends?*
4. Self-perception *Did you worry about your appearance?*	9. School *Were you satisfied with your school?*
5. Independence *Could you decide about your free time?*	10. Bullying *Did somebody ridicule you?*

The instrument assesses either the frequency of behavior/feelings or intensity of an attitude using a five-point Likert scale (1 = never, 2 = seldom, 3 = sometimes, 4 = often, 5 = always) The score for each dimension was transformed to a 0 to 100 point scale with higher scores indicate better HRQoL.

The Kidscreen instruments are available in child and adolescent as well as parent versions and have been translated and adapted for use in several languages. A score can be calculated and t-values and percentages will be available for each country stratified by age and gender.

The aims of the questionnaire is a diagnose of deterioration of a child's wellbeing as well as an identification of social and behavioural determinants of health. The practical purpose was to create a base for early intervention.

Resilience as a process

Research on resilience as a process treats it as an ability that develops over time as a result of interaction between an individual and his/her environment. The model developed by Constantine et al. demonstrates the way resilience in children is being shaped by certain external conditions. The following overview of children's resilience assets has been provided in The Healthy Kids Resilience Assessment (1999).

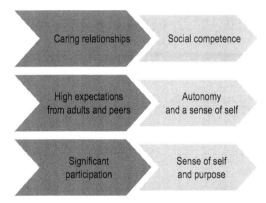

Figure 3. External and internal resources (as cited in Constantine et al., 1999)

These assets include social competence, defined as a capacity for effective communication, cooperation, empathy, responsibility and flexibility in social situations. An important role in this respect is played by caring and supportive relationships, that is, relationships with people who shape and foster the healthy development and well-being of a child. Thus, the quality of relationships within a family or an institution of early education proves to have a significant impact on the formation of children's social competence.

The next group of internal resources includes autonomy and a sense of self, defined as a sense of identity, internal power, self-efficacy and self-awareness. The external factors that influence the formation of this resource are high expectations from parents or peers. This means that if others believe that a child has the capacity to meet certain challenges, this can actually foster the development of his or her internal power and self-esteem.

The third group of internal resources comprises a sense of meaning and purpose, defined as an optimistic belief that one's life is coherent, purposeful and meaningful. A significant impact on the formation of this internal resource is made by significant and active participation, or participation in relevant, engaging and responsible activities. Stimulating factors in this respect are the chance to take responsibility and making one's own contribution to specific projects and initiatives (Constantine et al., 1999).

The theoretical model presented above combines two major areas that have been studied in various configurations in connection to resilience. It highlights the importance of external resources for the formation of resilience in children and provides a thorough description of the interdependence between internal and external resources vital for resilience.

The Healthy Kids Survey (HKS) is one of the few large-scale surveys to assess both risk and resilience. The HKS is a comprehensive student self-report tool connected with students' health. The survey's Resilience and

Youth Development Module (RYDM) is based on the premise that youth who experience high levels of environmental assets in three areas – high expectations from adults, caring relationships with adults, and opportunities for meaningful participation – will develop the resilience traits, the connection to school, and motivation to learn that lead to positive academic, social, and health outcomes (Constantine, Benard, Diaz, 1999).

In California an average of about 600,000 students take the Healthy Kids Survey and a part of the resilience and youth development module every year. The tool is mandated (since fall 2003) by the California Department of Education for compliance with No Child Left Behind and state Tobacco Use Prevention and Education (TUPE) grants.

Table 3 presents The Healthy Kids Survey in the elementary school version. External (environmental) resilience assets are divided into three groups of factors: school, home and peers. Internal resilience assets involve three factors: empathy, problem solving, goals and aspirations. There is one sample question presented for each field.

Table 3. Elementary school resilience and youth development module items by construct (after Hanson, Kim, 2007)

Environmental resilience assets, school assets	Sample Item
Caring relationships at school	Do the teachers and other grown-ups at school care about you?
High expectations at school	Do the teachers and other grown-ups at school believe that you can do a good job?
Meaningful participation at school	Do you do things to be helpful at school?
Environmental resilience assets, home assets	
Caring relationships at home	Does a parent or some other grown-up at home listen to you when you have something to say?
High expectations at home	Does a parent or some other grown-up at home want you to do your best?
Meaningful participation at home	Do you help out at home?
Environmental resilience assets, peer assets	
High expectations with peers	Do your best friends get into trouble?
Internal resilience assets	
Empathy	Do you try to understand how other people feel?
Problem-solving	Do you know where to go to get help with a problem?
Goals and aspirations	Do you have goals and plans for the future?

Possible responses include (1) no, never, (2) yes, some of the time, (3) yes, most of the time, (4) yes, all of the time.

The main aim of The Healthy Kids Survey is monitoring the school environment and student health risks. It was designed as an epidemiological surveillance tool to track aggregate levels of health risk and resilience.

The Healthy Kids Survey version for secondary school involves more constructs connected with internal resilience assests as: cooperation and communication, self-efficacy, self-awareness. Within Environmental resilience assets there is one additional construct namely community assets (with subscales caring relationship in community, high expectations in community, meaningful participation in community).

Both surveys (for elementary and secondary school) ought to answer the question how to measure resilient traits in children and young people and how to determine the role of the school environmental in promoting these traits (Constantine, Benard, Diaz, 1999; Hanson, Kim, 2007).

Resilience as an individual resource

"Resilience can be understood as an individual abillity crucial in coping and adaptation processes" (Ogińska-Bulik, Juczyński, 2011, p. 14).

The presented theoretical proposal is connected with person-focused studies of resilience. This approach attempts to grasp the configural patterns of adaptation like classification system for mental disorder and seeks to identify groups with good versus poor coping and adaptation abilities (Masten, 2001; Ogińska-Bulik, Juczyński, 2011; Kolar, 2011). Individual assets treated as protective factors have been researched in the ego-resiliency wave (the term was firstly proposed by Block in his non-published doctorthesis in 1950). Ego-resiliency means a general individual characteristics, abillity to modulate of ego control in order to maintain or strengthen homeostase in the system (Zwoliński, 2011). Within individual assets the following are listed: temperamental and cognitive factors, selfesteem, coping strategies, life approach, sense of meaning and purpose, factors important for social acceptation (Pilecka, Fryt, 2011).

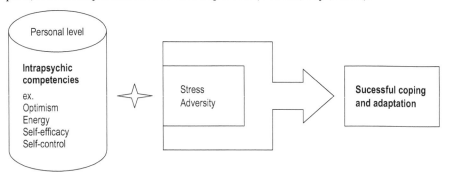

Figure 4. Model of individual assets

The first group of tools are observation scales completed by parents, carers and teachers, including the DECA, namely the Devereux Early Childhood Assessment (LeBuffe, Naglieri, 1998) or the DESSA, namely the Devereux Student Strengths Assessment (LeBuffe, Naglieri, Shapiro, 2006).

The DECA Assessment

The Devereux Early Childhood Assessment for Infants and Toddlers (LeBuffe, Naglieri, 1998) describes a child in standard version (37 items) or in the clinical version (62 items) in 4 dimentions as:

- Initiative

(ability to use independent thought and action to meet individual needs)

Self-control

- (ability to experience a range of feelings and express them in the social acceptable way)
- Attachment

(mutual, strong, long-lasting relationship between a child and significant adult)

- Problem behaviour

Two types of standard scores are provided for each child: percentiles and T-scores.

Children's results in protective factors (initiative, self-control and attachment) that fall one or more standard deviations above the mean are treated as "strengths" (T score – 60 or more. As "concerns" are classified children with results one or more standard deviations below the mean (T score – 40 or less). Children with results within one standard deviation (T score – 41–59) are called "typical."

In the DECA questionnaires parents and preschool teachers assess 5-year-old and younger children. The instrument was used very broadly in the HEAD START Project in the USA with a purpose to equalize school chance in children with disadvantaged life circumstances (Kordich Hall, 2010).

The questionnaire is involved in the DECA Program. The goals of this program are to identify young children's protective factors at home and school and to support parents and teachers to help each child strengthen his/her resilience. The third important purpose is to screen for children who may be exhibiting behavioral concerns before they develop behavioral disorders. Philosophy of the DECa Program underlines: "all children need resilience, not just children who are at-risk. Sometimes a tragedy, a natural disaster, a death in the family, a divorce, an illness, etc. comes up unexpectedly, which is when a child really needs to have strong protective factors and coping skills already in place" (LeBuffe, Naglieri, 1998, p. 14).

The DESSA Assessment

The Devereux Student Strengths Assessment (LeBuffe, Naglieri, Shapiro, 2006) diagnoses resilience in 8 sub-scales (72 items) by assessing socio-emotional key competencies in children in the age 5–14. The DESSa is a standardized, norm-referenced behaviour rating scale. The assessment can be completed by parents, teachers, school staff, social servies. For each of the items, the rater is asked to indicate on five-point-scale how often the child engaged in each activity over the past 4 weeks (teachers and both parents).

The skills connected with resilience resources are:

- self-awareness;
- social awareness;
- self-management;
- goal-directed behaviour;
- interpersonal skills;
- personal responsibility;
- decision making;
- and optimistic thinking.

Results show that the DESSA can differentiate between students with and without social, emotional and bahavioural problems. "The scales on the DESSA can be considered protective factors within a risk and resilience theoretical framework. High scores on DESSA scales were associated with significantly fewer behavioral problems for students at both high and average levels of risk" (Kordich Hall, 2010, p. 3). Both questionnaires (DECA and DESSA) are used not only for diagnostic purposes. They are involved in the protective and preventive programs. Results can be summarized for individual child and also for all children in the classroom. They have been developed as a part of a comprehensive program to foster the healthy social and emotional development of children.

The second group of measurement instruments are self reports. Young people answer the questions and describe their individual reactions and feelings.

Resilience Scale for Children and Youth-SPP 18

As an example Resilience Scale for Children and Youth-SPP 18 (Ogińska-Bulik, Juczyński, 2011) can be given. The test based on self-reporting methodology is designed for young people in the age of 12–18. The SPP 18 includes 18 items in 4 issues:

- Optimistic approach and energy;
- Perseverance and determination in action;
- Sense of humor and openness to new experiences;
- Personal competencies and tolerance of negative affect.

Table 2. Factors and sample items in the Resilience Scale for Children and Youth (Ogińska-Bulik, Juczyński, 2011)

Issue	Sample items
1. Optimistic approach and energy	*Despite adversities and difficulties I find life exciting*
2. Perseverance and determination in action	*I usually go straight to the purpose*
3. Sense of humor and openness to new experiences	*In everything I do I try to find positives*
4. Personal competencies and tolerance of negative affect	*I have enough energy to do what I have to do*

Possible answers are: 0 – definitely not, 1 – rather not, 2 – hard to tell, 3 – rather yes, 4 – definitely yes. Higher score means higher resilience. Sten scale describes score 1–4 as low resilience level, score 5–6 as average and 7–10 as high resilience level.

In the Polish research group (N = 332) there were found following results: a low resilience level – 31,3%, an average resilience level – 37,9% and high resilience level – 33,8%. (Ogińska-Bulik, Juczyński, 2011).

The authors propose using the scale for prediction of possible child's or teenager's reaction to critical life event, chronic disease in the family. The application of SPP 18 can have a positive influence on adaptation and help to monitor recovery processes.

Why it is important to identify resilience

Resilience is not an inborn personal quality and it develops over time. Early childhood plays a particularly important role in the development of resilience. Research on mental health shows that resilience is a dynamic quality that children develop in interaction with persons from their closest environment and through positive experience they derive as they solve problems and overcome difficulties. As regards positive attitude to both overcoming crises and obstacles and undertaking developmental tasks, the process of climbing from one educational level to the other, which in itself is conducive to further development, remains of critical importance in this respect (e.g. starting preschool or school education) (Benson, Leffert, Scales, Blyth, 1998; Froehlich-Gildhoff, Doerner, Roennau, 2007).

Developmental tasks that have been already completed form a basis for accomplishing further tasks. In the process, children acquire skills and competencies necessary for normal development. Effective coping implies further development and personal growth. Thus, children learn to treat changes and stressful situations as a challenge to meet (Wustmann, 2004; Petermann et al., 2004).

Enhancing resilience in children can be realized in the proactive approach, where children, parents and teachers are involved in many common actions (Alvord, Grados, 2005).

By recognizing the component competencies of what is known as life skills one can form a basis for introducing activities which stimulate the development of one's individual resources and which may also be used as programs that develop these competencies in preschool children. Such programs treat children as active achievers and co-creators of their own lives.

Thus, it can be defined as an attempt to instil resilience in children and adolescents through prevention, intervention and creating a protective system on the basis of the analysis of the current situation as well as current needs (as-is analysis). An important role in this respect may be played by institutions of preschool and early education which may help foster resilience resources in children. (Werner, Smith, 1992; Wyman et al., 1999). Empowering children and young people is the best way to give them some kind "key for health" (Froehlich-Gildhoff, Doerner, Roennau, 2007; Ogińska-Bulik, Juczyński, 2011).

References

Alvord, M.K., Grados, J.J. (2005). Enhancing Resilience in Children: A Proactive Approach. *Professional Psychology: Research and Practice*, 36, 3, 238–245.

Ames, E.W. (1997). *The development of Romanian orphanage children adopted to Canada (Final report to the National Welfare Grants Program: Human Resources Development Canada)*. Burnaby, British Columbia, Canada: Simon Fraser University.

Benson, P.L., Leffert, N., Scales, P.C., Blyth, D.A. (1998). Beyond the "village" rhetoric: Creating healthy communities for children and adolescents. *Applied Developmental Science*, 2 (3), 138–159.

Constantine, N., Benard, B., Diaz, M. (1999). Measuring protective factors and resilience traits in youth: The Healthy Kids Resilience Assessment. *American Psychologist*, 55, 647–654.

Froehlich-Gildhoff, K., Doerner, T., Roennau, M. (2007). *Praevention and Resiliencefoerderung in Kindertagseinrichtungen*. Muenchen, Basel: Ernst Reinhardt.

Garmezy, N. (1993). Children in poverty: Resilience despite risk. *Psychiatry* 1993, 56.

Garmezy, N. (1971). Vulnerability research and the issue of primary prevention. *American Journal of Orthopsychiatry*, 41, 101–116.

Goodman, R. (1997). The Strengths and Difficulties Questionnaire: A research note. *Journal of Child Psychology and Psychiatry*, 38, 581–86.

Hanson, T.L., Kim, J.O. (2007). *Measuring resilience and youth development: the psychometric properties of the Healthy Kids Survey.* (Issues, Answers Report, REL 2007 – No. 034). Washington, DC: U.S. Department of Education, Institute of Education Sciences, National Center for Education Evaluation and Regional Assistance, Regional Educational Laboratory West. Retrieved from http://ies.ed.gov/ncee/edlabs (2013).

Klein, J.D., Sabaratnam, P., Auerbach, M.M., Smith, S.M., Kodjo, C., Lewis, C., Ryan, S., Dandino, C. (2006). Development and factor structure of a brief instrument to assess the impact of community programs on positive youth development: The Rochester evaluation of asset development for youth (READY) tool. *Journal of Adolescent Health*, 39, 252–260.

Klohnen, E. (1996). Conceptual Analysis and Measurement of the Constant of Ego-Resiliency. *Journal of Personality and Social Psychology*, 70, 5, 1067–7109.

Kolar, K. (2011). Resilience: Revisiting the Concept and its Utility for Social Research. *In J. Mental Health Addiction*, 9: 421–433.

Kordich Hall, D. (2010). *Toronto: The Child, Family Partnership*; http://www.reachinginreachingout.com/documents/APPENDIXE-AnnotatedCompendiumofResiliencemeasures-Nov17-10copyright.pdf (2013).

Laucht, M., Blomeyer, D., Coneus, K. (2000). *Self-productivity and Complementarities in Human Development*. *Mannheim Study of Children at Risk*. Bonn: IZA.

LeBuffe, P., Naglieri, J., Shapiro, V. (2006). Devereux Foundation (www.studentstrengths.org).

LeBuffe, P., Naglieri, J. (1998). *Devereux Foundation, Early Childhood Initiative*, www.devereux.org (2013).

Leitpold, B., Greve, B. (2009). Resilience. A conceptual Bridge Between Coping and Development. *European Psychologist*, 14(1), 40–50.

Luthar, S.S. (1991) Vulnerability and resilience: A study of high-risk adolescents. *Child Development*, 62, 600–616.

Malmberg, L.E., Flouri, E. (2011). The comparison and interdependence of maternal and paternal influences on young children's behavior and resilience. *Journal of Clinical Child and Adolescent Psychology*, 50(3), 434–444.

Masten, A.S., O'Connor, M.J. (1998). Vulnerability, stress, and resilience in the early development of a high risk child. *J. Am. Acad. Child. Adolesc. Psychiatry*, March, 28 (2), 274–278.

Masten, A. (2001). Ordinary Magic. Resilience Process in Development. *American Psychologist*, 56, 3, 227–238.

Masten, A., Obradović, J. (2006). Competence and Resilience in Development. *Ann. N.Y. Acad. Sci.*, 1094, 13–27.

Mazur, J., Małkowska-Szkutnik, A., Dzielska, A., Tabak, I. (2008). *Polska wersja kwestionariuszy do badania jakości życia związanej ze zdrowiem dzieci i młodzieży (KIDSCREEN)*. Warszawa: Instytut Matki i Dziecka.

Mazur, J., Tabak, I. (2008). Koncepcja resilience. Od teorii do badań empirycznych. *Medycyna Wieku Rozwojowego* 2, cz. I, t. XII, 569–577.

Murphy, L.B, Moriarty, A. (1976). *Vulnerability, coping, and growth: From infancy to adolescence*. New Haven: Yale University Press.

Ogińska-Bulik, N., Juczyński, Z. (2011). Prężność u dzieci i młodzieży; charakterystyka i pomiar – polska skala SPP-18. *Polskie Forum Psychologiczne*, t. 16, 1, 7–28.

Olsson, C.A. et al.,(2003). Adolescent resilience: a concept analysis. *Journal of Adolescence*, 26, 1–11.

Ostaszewski, K., Borucka, A. (2008). Koncepcja resilience. Kluczowe pojęcia i wybrane zagadnienia. *Medycyna Wieku Rozwojowego* 2, cz. I, t. XII, 587–599.

Petermann, F. et al. (2004). *Entwicklungwissenschaft – Entwicklungspsychologie: Genetik-Neuropsychologie*. Berlin, Heidelberg: Springer.

Pilecka, W., Fryt, J. (2011). *Teoria dziecięcej odporności psychicznej*. [W:] W. Pilecka (Ed.). *Psychologia zdrowia dzieci i młodzieży. Perspektywa kliniczna*. Kraków: Wydawnictwo Uniwersytetu Jagiellońskiego, 48–68.

Riding, R., Rayner, S., Morris, S., Grimley, M., Adams, D. (2002). *Emotional and Behavioral Development Scales*. Birmingham, UK: Assessment Research Unit, School of Education, University of Birmingham.

Rutter, M. (1979) Protective factors in children's responses to stress and disadvantage. [In:] Kent, M.W., Rolf, J.E. (Ed.). *Primary prevention in psychopathology: Social competence in children*, Vol. 8, Hanover: University Press of New England, 49–74.

Rutter, M. (2006). Implications of resilience concepts for scientific understanding. *Annals New York Academy of Science*, 1094, 1–12.

Szmigielska, B. (1996). *SPK-DP – Skala Poczucia Kontroli u Dzieci Przedszkolnych*. Warszawa: Pracownia Testów Psychologicznych Polskiego Towarzystwa Psychologicznego.

Taplin, M. (2011). Silent sitting – a cross-curricular tool to promote resilience. *International Journal of Children and Spirituality*, 16, 2, 75–96.

Tugade, M.M., Fredrikson, B.L., Feldman Barrett, L. (2004). Psychological resilience and positive emotional granulity: examining the benefits of positive emotions on coping and health. *Journal of Personality*, 72, 6.

Ungar, M., Liebenberg, L. (2009). Cross-cultural consultation leading to the development of a valid measure of youth resilience: the international resilience project. *Studia Psychologica*, 51 (2–3), 259–269.

Werner, E.E. (2000). Protective factors and individual resilience. [In:] J.P. Shonkoff, S.J. Meisels (Ed.). *Handbook of Early Childhood Intervention*. Second edition, USA: Cambridge University Press, 115–132.

Werner, E., Smith, R. (1992). *Overcoming the Odds: High-Risk Children from Birth to Adulthood*. New York: Cornell University Press.

Wustmann, C. (2004). *Resilienz: Widerstandsfaehigkeit von Kindern in Tageseinrichtungen foerdern*. Weinhaeim, Basel: Beltz.

Younkin, S.L., Betz, N.E. (1996). *Psychological hardiness: A reconceptualization and measurement*. [In:] T.W. Miller (Ed.). *Theory and assessment of stressful life events. International Universities Press stress and health series* (161–178). Madison, CT: International Universities Press.

Bogusława Piasecka, Krzysztof Gerc, Iwona Sikorska
Jagiellonian University
Institute of Applied Psychology

SIBLINGS – A RETROSPECTIVE ANALYSIS OF DEIDENTIFICATION PROCESSES

Abstract

The article presents the analysis of interviews with adults who recall their relations with siblings. Differentiation processes are taken into consideration with a particular concern. Deidentification processes determine how siblings, especially of the same gender, develop individual characteristics, sense of identity in interests, views and manner. The theoretical background to the conducted study is F.F. Schachter's (1976, 1978) concept and W. Toman's (1961) theory of family constellations considering the connections between birth order and personality traits. F.F. Schachter's deidentification concept concerns which sibling pairs differ the strongest and presents developmental function of this process.

Key words: siblings, family constellations, deidentification processes, identification, rivalry

Introduction

Cain and Abel, Antigone and Polynices, Hansel and Gretel, Kai and Gerda are sibling archetypes which have placed in world culture and survived in people's consciousness. They are examples of emotionally multicoloured relations between siblings, there can be found care, love, devotion, conflict, jealousy and so extreme envy that might be fatal. They let us become familiar with these emotions in real brother-sister relations. Research on family usually considers pairs parents-children or parents. Siblings have been neglected, the influence of relations between brothers and sisters on their later friendship and intimate relationship was undervalued. Psychoanalysts make much of a contribution to conceptualize brother-sister relationships (Walewska, 2011). The First International

Conference of Two Section of the European Federation for Psychoanalytic Psychology with the title "Siblings, Rivalry and Envy – Coexistence and Concern" took place in Kraków in 2011. The presented papers[1], mainly based on clinical research, raised the most important aspects of siblings relations and coincided with other research, not only psychoanalytic paradigm. The most common subjects described in the psychology literature are the reaction of the older sibling to the appearance of the younger one, impairment, sibling incest (Bank, Kahn, 1997), the loss of sibling (Pantke, Slade, 2006) and the moderating role of parents and other adults in creating relations between sibling (Piotrowski, 2011; Schachter et al., 1976, 1978). The problems and conflicts in families are coherent with the issues reported by psychological practitioners. Among theories concerning developmental regularities of sibling relation, the A. Goetting's (1986) theory describing developmental tasks at successive stages of family development and frequently quoted W. Toman's (1961) theory of family constellations are noteworthy. A. Goetting determines sibling tasks, which changes with the family development. A sister is a playmate and brother may give the emotional support in childhood and in adolescence children solidarity facilitates restructuring of the family system, thereby it creates favourable conditions for the family development. Sibling relationships constitute the training for cooperation, sharing, loyalty and separation.

In adulthood siblings may help each other, give advice in their parenthood and later share the care of ageing parents. W. Toman's conception assumes that children are trained specific standards of behaviour on the basis of their birth order. The older siblings are demanded to be protective towards their younger brother or sisters and more responsible and mature. While the younger siblings develop adaptive skills and tendency to carefree behaviour. In 1976 F.F. Schachter with team published their findings of the survey interviews on sibling similarities and differences. The respondents were undergraduates from two- or three-child families. The questionnaire, consisted of four parts, concerned the assessment of the level of identification and diversification between respondents and their siblings. One part of the questionnaire examined the retrospective evaluation of parents' attitude towards respondents' siblings. The research results prove that in two-child families the level of deidentification – differentiation is high regardless of children gender, but in thee-child families the highest level of deidentification was between the first and the second child of the same sex, the second-highest level was observed between the first and the third child. The intermediate level of deidentification was between the second and the third child. Deidentification facilitates taking up different activities, enables the development of separate interests and predestinates to individuation. Interpreting the general findings, the authors referred to psychoanalytic theories and proposed a thesis,

---

[1] Conference materials, EFPP, PTPP Conference, Kraków 2011.

that deidentification is a mechanism that simplifies solving sibling rivalry and consequently Cain complex.

Similar conclusions were reached by the team of researchers under F.F. Schachter's direction (1978). The study in which mothers gave their opinion about their children, enriched the conception of parental contribution in weakening or strengthening the deidentification process. Parents through delegation processes (Stierlin, 1998) or parental projection (Bowen, after Goldenberg, Goldenberg, 2006) influence relations between sibling intensifying or calming rivalry. Gabbard's (2010) theory suggests taking into consideration complementarity and temperamental symmetricalness in family relation between a parent and child. The above conclusions let us debunk the myth of treating all children in family equally. The 'misfit' or 'unselected' child feels less loved by parents what is very often reinforced by another important people from outside the nuclear family (cf. Joyce, 2011). Not only parents 'choose' children, siblings do the same, in large families siblings pair up. S.P. Bank and M.D. Kahn (1997) describe it in a thorough analysis of sibling relations based on the psychotherapeutic work experience with individuals and families. Pairing up expressed by more frequent shared games or activities and greater loyalty is not connected with gender and age similarity but developing personality traits. Mostly the first and the third child pair up, these pairs have lower level of rivalry than between the first and the second child.

Since the dawn of time rivalry is a part of relations between brothers and sisters. J. Mittchel (Walewska, 2011) considers that appearance of an infant, which takes older sibling's place and becomes a rival, as a threat to complete loss of parents' love and rejection of the older child for the new one. Similarly, the second and every next child in family have no access to the blissful times of parents and the first-born triangle, hence they may feel isolated and excluded from family.

Children continuously compete for attention, favour and parent's recognition and they cope with the frustration of not being just one.

Parents may neutralize anxiety and frustration through containing, thereby they soothe rivalry, jealousy and envy. On the other hand, sibling means having mutual care, identification object, and structuralizing inner child's word and supportive development influence (Cole, 2011; Whitman et al., 2007). Sibling relations facilitate the process of forming interpsycholgical and intrapsychological personality, the relations enable them to experience the mutuality and exchange, the fight and forgiveness.

Siblings make important objects of reference in psycho-sexual development (Bank, Kahn, 1997). Brother or sister is the first alike/different person in the face of whom the sexual identity develops. The first naked person that a child gets to know is usually its sibling, then the body is compared and the child learns the differences and similarities. Siblings may be the source of initial erotic experience for each other during sexual plays. Bank and Kahn describe the cases of crossing the bounds of sexual play between sibling and analyse the results of incest on the further psychosexual development of the children and their partnership in adulthood. Incest occurred when children felt neglected by parents.

The relations with sibling also influence the development of children's resilience. The model of internal and external resources shaping the resilience of individuals (Constantine et al., 1999) indicates that the value and course of the sibling relationship may make so-called external assets which form the internal assets, that is high self-esteem, autonomy, sense of meaning and purpose in actions. Enriching the internal assets enhance the ability of an individual to regain the balance after hard and sometimes traumatic experiences and its competence to protect, self-appease and repair.

It can be established that sibling relations are the base for partnership, friendship and the position in a group. Thanks to relations with a brother or sister the child has a chance to acquire the ability to tolerate other people and their dissimilarity. In everyday sibling relations the need for assimilation and differentiation forms at the same time.

Method

This study concerns the sibling relations form the perspective of adults. The aim of the research is to describe and understand the processes of deidentification – separation from brother or sister and development of individual characteristic.

There were constructed two research questions at the stage of planning:

1. How are sibling relations shaped within the space of successive developmental stages.
2. How does deidentification process proceed between siblings.

The subjects were people from different positions in family constellations to obtain the point of view of the relation of older sister, older brother and younger sister and younger brother. The authors selected people recommended by their acquaintances, who agreed to take part in the research and gave their phone numbers. The research was conducted in April and May 2011, in the form of free form tape-recorded interviews lasted 60 to 90 minutes. The subjects were informed about the topic of the conversation, that is *We're going to ask you about relations with your siblings*. The duration of interviews was dependent on the openness and candidness of each subject. After the fieldwork, the transcription of the interviews was accomplished. The transcribed material was read to select the main topics, then the material form all interviews was collected with reference to the main topics. The selected topics were entitled: main characters, the earliest memory, deidentification, rivalry, care and play, psychosexual development.

The interviews analysis

The following analysis contains numerous quotations from the subjects. The quotations are written in italics. The anonymity of subjects is remained in order to prevent from their identification. Four people were interviewed, they are marked with capital letters MM1, MD2, KE1, KN2 in this paper.

Main characters

The subjects, their sibling and parents are presented below. MM1 is a 36-year-old man, having higher education in arts. He is married with no children and he is an older brother in his family of origin. His sister is 32, she is married with three children. She does not work, she is a housewife. She has secondary education.

MM1's father is 63, he has higher education. He was a teacher but he took early retirement. MM1's mother is 60, she has secondary education and still works. The subject has a good relationship with his family of origin. When he meets his sister they *always have a lot to talk about*. MM1 found the proposal for an interview on relations with sister interesting, and he span the tale spontaneously just after the introductory question.

The next subject is MD2, a 31-year-old man with higher technical education but he does not work in his field. He is in the service sector. He is married with no children. His wife graduated in psychology and work as an educational psychologist. MD2 is the middle child in his family of origin, he has 32-year-old brother and 22-year-old sister. His brother is married and he has a small child. The brother, as the only one in the family, has secondary education and *never applied himself to his studies and did not want to enter university.* The MD2's sister is an undergraduate and lives with parents. MD2's parents have secondary education and are in the service sector. His father is 57 and mother is 62. MD2 describes the relations with his brother as conflictive, similarly to relations with his father. They do not meet very often. Family parties usually ends with a row. He has very good relations with his sister and mother. The subject described his family of origin spontaneously and freely.

KE1 is a 25-year-old woman with higher pedagogic education but she works off and on as a waitress or receptionist. She is the youngest child in her family of origin. She did not start a family and she is not in a matrimonially oriented relationship either. Her older sister is 31, she has a partner and a small son. She has secondary education. Another sister is 29, she has university education. She is married with two daughters. She said her father is *unknown*. Their mother died when KE1 was five. The three girls were brought up by their grandparents, their mother's parents. The subject spoke about her parents perfunctorily and reluctantly, whereas she talked a lot about her sisters, especially the oldest one, who she has very close relations with. More detailed questions had to be asked during the interview because KE1's statements were laconic. KE1's non-verbal signals signified her emotional agitation, thus the interviewer talked over KE1's state. KE1 said she was fine and wanted to continue the conversation.

KN2 is a 83-year-old woman, a sister of a deceased brother. She has not completed higher medical education. When she was 70 she stopped working. She has been a widow for ten years. She has a son and daughter, two grandsons, two granddaughters and two great-granddaughters. Her brother was two years older, he had higher education. He was married with a son. Their parents had vocational secondary education, their father died at the age of 80 and mother at the age of 77. At the beginning KN2 was doubtful whether the interview with her will be useful. With the unfolding conversation, she become more spontaneous and it was visible that evoking her memories pleased her (she smiled and she went into detail). At the end, she thanked for *the trip to her childhood.*

The earliest memory

Every interview was started with a question about the earliest memory connected with brother or sister and it was the invitation to bring the childhood back at the same time. The older brothers remember the moment when their parents told them that they were expecting a baby. MM1 and Md2 could describe the situation in detail.

MM1 was four when his parents told them that there would be another baby in the family. He did not remember his emotional answer but the thought of having sibling was with him *always.*

MD1: *When my sister was born, I grew accustomed to her, I took care of her.* MM1 remembers his sister as *a powerhouse of energy.* She was full of ideas and always ready for experimentation.

MD2 remembers the conversation with his mother and father about the expected sister. Parents told him, an 11-year-old boy, and his a year older brother about their sister just before labour. Both brothers were astonished and they said: *we're so old and there will be a baby? When parents brought her home I kissed her feet and hands, we were pleased. We were taking care of here, my brother even could replace the nappy of her. I was afraid of hurting her but he wasn't.* MD1 remembers his brother as a boy who is afraid of nothing, *a daredevil, and a pugnacious boy who always achieved what he wanted.* They still have the picture of the sister as a little girl demanding care and help.

KE1 evoked the childhood memories with difficulty. *I've never thought about it, I remember it indistinctly.* After a few minutes of silence she recalled about a happening during breakfast when she was five or six and her middle sister *poured chocolate over her head. I couldn't wash it in the shower.* The subject talked very little about her early childhood, she remembers better her past from adolescence. She remembers her middle sister as a swaggering tomboy who had her own life and the oldest sister as a candid girl and remembering about others.

The first KN2 memory is when she was three or four: *mum was looking for us, she was calling and spread her arms so that we were running to her and hugged.* She also remembers a visit at her family's when she was five or six and together with her two-year-older brother teased their younger cousin, who provoked them, *he hit and pushed us because he was jealous so we integrated against him.* KN2 was interested in everything what her brother did: *I was stalking and imitating him.* What she remembers very well from her childhood was the constant conflict between her father and brother which was present for all their lives.

Care and play

Two interviews were conducted with the representatives of two children families, and another two with the representatives of three children families.

MM1 is an older brother, KN2 is a younger sister. In MM1's family there is a four year gap between sibling, between KN2 and her deceased brother was two years difference. The older brother describing the relations with her sister when she was an infant emphasized the role of his parents who directed his behaviour towards his sister:

MM1: *parents gave such a space so I could feed my little sister or drive her pram and play with her in the way I could. They taught me not to hurt her.*

When MM1 was of primary school age she watched TV with her sister: *At first it was a black-and-white TV set, then colour. I was sitting on the sofa bed and my sister, the powerhouse of energy, was watching the TV upside down. She had her legs on the wall and she even provoked me, it was charming and pleasant.*

Their bonds loosened when MM1 reached his adolescence. He remember keeping distance, but when his sister reached her adolescence their relation strengthened again. Their parents delegated him to talk with sister about contacts *with boys.* The subject described these conversations *as a turning point in our relation, these talks bound us, we had our secrets.* He finds the currents relations with sister very close and full of positive emotions. They give mutual support to each other:

When I have some difficulties in relations with my wife, I text to my sister and when she is at the party and doesn't want to get back on her own she doesn't call either her husband or our father but she calls me. She's dear to my heart. I have the sister with the same blood type and eyes colour. When our parents are not here, I'll have her.

KN2 remembers from her and her two-year-old brother childhood reading of books and listening to family stories told by their mother. They attended primary school and their free time they spent at home. KN2 evoked the memory of playing chess with her brother and a scene of going with him to a teacher who they borrowed books from.

The lady had a beautiful edition of Rodziewiczówna and Kraszewski collection. We're running to her holding each other by the hand. She lent us two books every time and we gave them back.

KN2 told their parents attached importance to their schooling what her brother disregarded. Her brother *got poor marks so their father engaged private tutors, one went in and another went out. My brother couldn't stand it, he left the house for a moment and ran around it, then he knocked at my window and broke the window. He pleaded not guilty.*

The subject told that parent wanted her to quiz him on Latin vocabulary. They were trained to study and work. KN2 helped her mother with housework. *Father kept her brother on the go, either he had to study or do even ridiculous things as nails straightening.*

KN2's and her brother adolescence coincided with World War II. She talked about the flight from the war at the very first days and about bombing raids and the danger and anxiety which were present all the time: *the anxiety brought us closer together.* According to the occupying force law children were forced to work from the age of 14. KN2 worked in a shoe shop and her brother in a chemical laboratory. After the war they joined the scouts, they had mutual friends and the first love affairs. After school-leaving examinations her brother went to college and she was interested in his studies: *I attended the lectures with him. He asked me to be quiet and not to look at the lecturer in order to be unnoticed.*

In adulthood their relations were diversified, the phases of closeness alternated with loosening of their bonds and isolation. At the end of his life they brought closer. KN2 emphasized that she took care of him from their childhood.

The two following interviews were conducted with the younger sister (KE1) of three sisters and the middle brother (MD2) of the siblings of two brothers and a sister.

There is one year age difference between MD2 and his older brother.

MD2: *Parents treated us as twins. Although we didn't go to school together, we made our First Communion in the same time. They enrolled us on the same extra classes, we kept close together. We were naughty children, we had risky ideas so we were punished in the same way. We played together in the courtyard and we had the same friends.*

By his accounts, peer and similarly their parents did not differentiate them: when one quarrelled with somebody, the other got a beating as well.

They enhanced their inseparability through loyalty and mutual help: *we were at one with each other at trainings. Arguments and fights broke out between them at the same time: we were always fighting but I don't remember why, probably because of bullshit. When the sister was born they tried to be gentle with her what their parents kept an eye on.* The subject remember being angry with her: *I punched her doll. When she was 16, I was taking her to parties. I treated her seriously, but our brother – patronizingly. She has better contact with me now, than with our brother. She helps at my company, she substitutes me. She's reliable.* Current relations between the brothers are conflictual, they tried to run a company but they split up after a raw and *ruck*.

KE1 told us several times that she remembers very little about her children. Her family situation is special, after she was born her parents split up and her mother died when KE1 was five. Her mother's parents brought up her and her two sisters. There is a two year age gap between the older sisters and they *stuck together, separately from me. They didn't look after me, only my grandma did it. They went out together and I stayed with my grandma.* The subject said: *as the youngest one I was protected by my grandparents, their favourite, they were overprotective.* When she was a teenager the sisters took her to the swimming pool, cycling or roller-skating, but she had to be self-reliant. When they reached their adolescence: *they avoided me.* In adulthood KE1 brought closer to her sisters, especially the oldest one, *we're very close now, although she lives abroad, we're very much alike and we differ from our middle sister.* KE1 describes the oldest sister as protective and loving person and KE1 responds her in the same way. She worries about her sister: *whether she doesn't work too much, she should have some time only for herself.* The middle sister *lives her own life*, the subject emphasized her dissimilarity and the distance she keeps, although they live close to each other.

Rivalry

Jealousy in sibling relations was mentioned in all interviews. There was jealousy of presents, own room (MM1), toys, *who's got a better bike, who's got more money* (KE1), availability of education (KN2). In all cases of sibling rivalry, an important role was played by adults from family and social environment. MM1 quoted the example of comparing him to his sister at school by teachers. He had indeed been given to her as the example of more diligent student, but he remembers: *she does nothing, she doesn't study at home but she knows more.* He had the feeling of being burdened more with housework: *I was beating dust out of carpets, and vacuuming, but she did nothing.* There was a division in MM1's family: *mother's son and father's daughter. When I was 15 and she was 12 we fight and she smashed his lip, she was punished by our mother.* It was obvious for him and their parents that he as the older one should have had his own room. His sister had a connecting room what was the cause of countless quarrels. She felt she was treated unfairly.

KN2 remembers that her parents blatantly favoured her brother, *he was always put first, his son is the eighth wonder of the world to our mother.* The subject implied that education was very important in her family of origin. Parents, especially her father, motivated her brother to study: *our father really wanted my brother to play the violin, he event bought him a violin but he wasn't successful in convincing him.* KN2 remembers a conversation with her father after she passed the secondary school-leaving examinations: *it was very hard, my brother was studying, my father told me "you've already passed your exams, think what you've achieved."* She begun work: *my mother fixed me up with the office job.* When KN2 was asked about her emotions connected with the happenings she told about sadness and envy. She thinks that envy appears later, when she was adult or when she started her family and had children. In KN2's family of origin it was obvious that her brother had a privileged position: *they showed leniency towards him, and he expected the same from me. He used my help, he borrowed from me, being precisely, he took my things. My mother was lenient towards him and she helped him more than me.*

KE1 describing the rivalry between sisters told that they were competing *for everything, we were quarrelling, there wasn't such a thing as sharing. We were quarrelling about money, they were given notes but I was given coins and I was pleased that it was more than they had.* The older sisters did not let her enter their society: *they had secrets from me, I felt hurt.* Grandmother and grandfather, who brought the girls up after their parents' death, repeated over and over again that *everything must be justly and shared evenly.* KE1 thinks that they favoured her as the youngest of the three sisters. They protected her excessively and forgave everything to compensate for the loss of her mother. The subject envied her sisters the freedom and similar rights but she only heard: *when you're at their age, we'll let you do that.*

MD2 emphasized the closeness with his brother at the beginning of the conversation, then he was requested to present their psychological characteristics. He described his brother a truculent, reckless boy who is open-minded and sociable. While he presented himself as a prudent, cautious and introverted person. He finds his brother used him: *his motorbike was always broken so he was taking mine.* They practiced judo from their early childhood and they fought at home as well: *we beat each other continuously*, but he added immediately: *we stuck together.* The subject mentioned about the intergenerational approach, which was cultivated by his grandmother and maintained by his parents: *I was left out, the first-born is the most important.* Therefore, the family business was made over to his older brother who did not turn out to be a good businessman and misspent money: *he had four laptops and bought another one. Then, they acknowledged me.* The brothers ran the family business together for a while but then a conflict arose and the company collapsed.

Psychosexual development

MM1 remembers having baths with his sister in his early childhood and his discovery that their anatomies are different. The discovery was astonishing and fascinating.

MM1: *I think I was 8 when I decided not to bathe together with my sister.* He also remembered his admiration for the photo of his sister, she wore a white dress with blue flounces. MM1 did not want to talk about his matters with sister, but she tried to overstep the boundaries of intimacy. He satisfied his curiosity connected with sexuality by having conversations with his school friends: *I was curious what they feel during menstruation, but I talked about it with girls, my peers.* When MM1's sister became interested in boys: *I was jealous of her. I couldn't believe she formed a relationship with a guy. After she got married we started talking about men and women, it was a turning point.*

MD2 shared a room with his brother. Until we reached our adolescence, *we were fighting everyday just before we got into bed but when we were older we were talking about girls.* The subject talked about his involvement in intimate relationships of his sister: *I always wanted to get to know her boyfriends. When she said that a boy is proper, he probably was, but I wanted to check if he wasn't a cheat. During her teenage rebellion period she met a drug addict, I told her that he wasn't right for her. Parents didn't have to intervene.*

KE1 remembers the feeling of jealousy and the admiration for her sisters when they were getting ready for parties. She sat in the bathroom and watched how they put on their make-up or style their hair, at that time she wanted to join them. She dissociate herself form their choices now. KE1 does not talk with her sisters about *women's topics, I have a friend for that.*

When KE1's brother *was 12 or 13 he had a friend, she was a head taller than he. She was from our neighbourhood. He waited for her at the gate and they went to school together. I remember my surprise that such a beautiful, grown-up girl wanted to be friends with such a little grammar school pupil. When he fell in love with his wife-to-be, he wrote a memoir. He described there his feelings to Basia and I used to pilfer it and read.* Her brother was also interested in her life: *he didn't like when he saw me at school in boys' company. When a boy walked me home, he told our parents about it.* KN2 talked about a happening, which evoked an emotional stir: *my fiancé bought a book, it was the latest publication in Poland – "Ideal Marriage" by Van de Velde. When my brother saw it, he was furious and burnt the book. He fuelled a fire with the book. I was indignant with him, I wandered how he could butt in my affairs. We argued. At first he tore the pages out of the book and then he burnt it. I was somewhat under his influence and he was under the influence of the clergy so the book was sinful to him.*

Deidentification

The need for being different from brother or sister was described by all subjects, especially the subjects of the same-sex siblings emphasized their dissimilarity.

MD2 mentioned that his father put an accent on their physical fitness. They watched films with Bruce Lee and at the age of six they started practising judo. When they were 12 they had a fight during a workout: *it was a fist fight, I wiped the floor with him so I was expelled from the club. Then I started playing basketball.* The subject presented also the personality differences: *my brother forgets quickly but I feel bitter towards him. He's capable of getting mad but also easy to get appeased. I'm more conscientious. I was a good student. He dropped out of college. He bought a motorbike and had an accident. He embezzled money. He got married quickly and divorced after a year. I finished college. I have a wife. We live modestly. I'm a reliable person but my brother is a good-for-nothing. He is wasteful, I'm economical. He had short-term relationships but I'm in a long-term relationship.* MD2 described his feelings connected with the differences he mentioned above: *I envy him a little and perhaps I admire him for his lifestyle. He's always been carefree but I can't and I don't want to be like that.* When KE1 was asked about the similarities and differences between the three sisters she said she remembers little from her childhood. She brought the time back when her older sisters *started dying their hair and make themselves up, then I wanted to be like them.* At that time they separated from KE1, they had secrets and they went out together. Then the sisters started misbehaving, *I didn't want to distress my grandma, I didn't behaved badly. I used to put school first and now work is the most important thing for me.* The subject described also the differences between sisters in their adult lives: *we have different attitude to life. Unlike my sisters I always wanted to get an education first and then start a family. We have different friends, different clothes and likings.*

MD1 and KE1 also stressed the different approach to education of their siblings. Regardless of the birth order the subject showed themselves at their best. They saw themselves more submitted to parents or teachers and their brothers or sisters were shown as wayward rebels. MM1 found that *my sister rebelled for two of us. When she was 13 she didn't read required readings but "In Search of Lost Time." She was brave for me and showed me that there's another way of doing things. I was well-behaved and I helped with housework but she went out when she wanted. When she was given a trashing she said that she didn't give a monkey's about it and did what she wanted again. She was sociable but I was alone. She had fascination for people, I had fascination for music.* MM1 recalled that he was given more trust but less attention.

KN2 presented her brother similarly *as neglecting his school duties.* She sees herself as a submissive and reliable person. The subject said that her brother *wanted to influence my life. At that time men were more important, they were always right and parents also agreed with it. I wasn't the kind of a slave and I had my own conception of life.* She also described searching for the outlook on life by her brother: *the age of puberty was a fight, he started working in a laboratory and brought home the communist reasoning. My mother and me were horrified at what he was thinking. He rather provoked our father who was a great patriot being enamoured of Piłsudski.*

Discussion

The research was inspired by the questions about the shape and dynamics of sibling relations within the space of successive stages of development and the questions about the course of deidentification process.

The concept of deidentification and family constellations are the theoretical background. The concept of deidentification implies the existence of differentiation processes which are necessary for self-creation, while the family constellations theory describes how children are trained to behave according to definite patterns depending on the birth order. The interviews with adults and children and their retrospective stories revealed that a brother or sister are important people in their past and at presence in each case. The sibling relations changed with the developmental changes of adolescent participants of the relations (Goetting, 1986). In many cases the quality and dynamics of the sibling relations were created by people from family and social environment. The analysis of the interviews shows that older brothers remember very well the moment when they found out about the births of a new family member. On the basis of the described reactions, it can be assumed that the information about the future sister and the birth of her aroused strong emotions, positive e.g. tenderness towards the sister as well as negative – anger at parents (Walewska, 2011). By the subjects' accounts it can be stated that children were creators of the relations and the developing personalities were the moderating factors. The background to the relations were parents, grandparents and teachers – their values, beliefs and stereotypes concerning the rights and duties of gender or seniority and the social roles. A pattern of closeness and emotional distance between sibling is observed in most of the analysed cases. In the early childhood, especially when the age difference is insignificant, the closeness is expressed by mutual play, care and loyalty. The loosening of the bonds occurs when the older sibling reach their adolescence. Then the sibling bond strengthen again at puberty of the younger sibling. The loosening of the bonds helps to enter the close emotional relationships with people from outside family and prevents sibling incest (Bank, Kahn, 1997).

Siblings make a mutual potential for tension relief, including sexual tension and they also give each other the possibility to experience the relief resulting from the confirmation and recognition their desires. From what the subjects reported, it appears that siblings were interested in developmental changes and intimate life of their brothers or sisters. The observation and control were conducted secretly or openly. Older brothers were more active, they probably because of the cultural model took over the responsibility and right to interference in sisters' lives. The interference was expected to stop the development of relationship with people from outside the family but paradoxically, it could tighten contacts with these people and facilitate the sisters' separation in consequence. In all presented cases siblings were important points of reference in individuation and building autonomy processes. Referring to the subjects descriptions, it became clear that a brother or sister is the first and successive source of observations connected with the sameness and difference in appearance, temperament and personality. Sibling perform an important role in sexual identity formation, the sexual self. Mutual games and daily routines satisfy children's curiosity about thinking, feeling and behaving alike/different in comparison with their sibling. The sibling relationship help to obtain the reciprocal information on themselves. The psychological portraits of a brother or sister presented by the subjects are resultants of their feelings towards described sibling. If admiration, friendship and loyalty are present in the relationship, positive characteristics dominate in the sibling description. Similarly, if envy and regret are present, negative features are emphasized illustrated by examples. Ambivalent feelings also appears, e.g. jealousy or admiration for a taking risk brother or independent sister. It proves that the involvement in sibling relations is present in spite of the death or separation. Most of the subjects had vivid memories from very early ages except for a young woman who experienced trauma, she was abandoned by father and her mother died.

The background to sibling relations is family context. The regularity connected with roles assignment is observed, the roles are following: a responsible child and good-for-nothing, more or less dependent on parents' opinion obedient, and dutiful and a rebellious good-for-nothing. These roles are ascribed regardless of the age or gender what partly prove correct Toman's (1961) theory of training and reinforcing children in specific characteristics and consequently of behaviour patterns. The interviews show that ascription of roles to children is not connected with the birth order and gender but probably with personality predisposition of individual, parental projection and intergenerational transmission (Goldenberg, Goldenberg, 2006). Sibling paired up in the subjects' families of three children, what confirm Khan and Bank's research. The pairs may change throughout their childhood and adolescence and the choice is determined by age closeness in childhood and then by subjective similarity regardless of gender and age.

Irrespective of intensive rivalry between sibling, in this case – between brothers, the bonds with people from outside their family tighten and the loyalty to social context increased. The need for individuality is sometimes connected with opposition to cultural stereotypes. Identification processes alternate with rivalry that facilitates differentiation and consequently it shapes defining themselves.

Conclusions and implications

The study confirmed the importance of relations between sibling and their influence on development and functioning of children and then adults. The need for differentiation and identity emphasis is very strong, it motivates to rebel against family and cultural rules. The quality of sibling relations is moderated by the quality of the family relation, so it indicates the intensity of tension and conflicts, which can be reached by the relations between children. The findings might be applied in practice by family therapists and specialists in social security. Taking into consideration the above data it is recommended in therapy or other forms of help to give more attention to diagnose the sibling relationship. Directing attention to relations between children might help to understand the complexity of family problems and might make the prevention of such problems.

The relations between brothers and sisters might enrich internal resources of an individual and might also shape and increase the resilience of children, then adults. Drawing on the above conclusions, extensive literature and empirical experiences it is worth constructing a questionnaire diagnosing the relations between children in family. The questionnaire would complement the existing research methods.

References

Bank, S.P., Kahn, M.D. (1997). *The Sibling Bond.* New York: Basic Books.

Constantine, N., Benard, B., Diaz. M. (1999). Measuring protective factors and resilience traits in youth: The Healthy Kids Resilience Assessment. *American Psychologist*, 55, 647–654.

Gabbard, G.O. (2010). *Psychiatria psychodynamiczna w praktyce klinicznej.* Kraków: Wydawnictwo Uniwersytetu Jagiellońskiego.

Goetting, A. (1986). The developmental tasks of siblings over the life cycle. *J. Mar. Fam.*, 48, 703–714.

Goldenberg, H., Goldenberg, I. (2006). *Terapia rodzin.* Kraków: Wydawnictwo Uniwersytetu Jagiellońskiego.

Pantke, R., Slade, P. (2006). Remembered parenting style and psychological well-being in young adults whose parents had experienced early child loss. *The British Psychological Society, Psychology and Psychotherapy: Theory, Research and Practice*, 79, 69–81.

Piotrowski, C.C. (2011). Patterns of Adjustment Among Siblings Exposed to Intimate Partner Violence, Americ an Psychological Association. *Journal of Family Psychology*, Vol. 25, No. 1, 19–28.

Toman, W. (1961). *Family Constellation: Theory and Practice of a Psychological Game.* New York: Springer Publishing Company, INC.

Walewska, K. (2011). *Progi narodzin. Rola teorii w pracy psychoanalitycznej. Doświadczenia własne.* Kraków: Wydawnictwo Uniwersytetu Jagiellońskiego.

Whiteman, S.D., McHale, S.M., Crouter, A.C. (2007). The Pennsylvania State University Competing Processes of Sibling Influence: Observational Learning and Sibling Deidentification. *Blackwell Publishing Ltd. Social Development*, 16, 4, 642–661.

Klaus Fröhlich-Gildhoff, Maike Rönnau-Böse
Protestant University of Applied Sciences, Freiburg, Germany

EMPOWER CHILDREN! THE PROMOTION OF RESILIENCE IN EARLY CHILDHOOD INSTITUTIONS (KINDERGARTEN) AND PRIMARY SCHOOLS

Abstract

The following article presents the theoretical background, methods and evaluation re-sults of a practice research project to promote resilience in early childhood institutions. The project was financed by the German Ministry for Education and Research (BMBF 2008–2010) and takes a holistic and multidimensional approach by including profession-als, children, parents and networks of early childhood institutions. The project is based on the intervention programme "Empowering Children!" (ZfKJ, 2005–2007; Rönnau, Kraus-Gruner, Engel, 2008) and addresses ECI situated in areas with a high level of diversity (e.g. high percentage of immigrant families, high poverty levels, etc.). The pro-ject's goal is to empower these institutions to develop as target-group-oriented centres for mental health promotion from the resilience perspective. The results of the evaluation show positive effects on self-esteem, behavioural-stability and cognitive development of children who participated in the project (intervention group), in contrast to those identi-fied in a comparison group. The project's positive results lead to an enlargement and new approach: the promotion of life skills and resilience in primary schools.

Key words: early childhood education, prevention, resilience

Introduction

Mental health promotion and the perspective of resilience

Research and theory building of mental health and its promotion changed within the last 20 years from a deficit-orientated view to the analysis of the impor-tance of resources and protective factors. (e.g., Cicchetti, Cohen, 2006; Lösel,

Bender, 2007; Luthar, Cicchetti, 2000; Opp, Fingerle, 2007; Petermann, Nie-bank, Scheithauer, 2004; Werner, 2007). Influenced by long-term studies, especially the Kauai – longitudinal study (Werner, 1997, 2007), the concept of resilience – the ability to manage crises, difficult situations and developmental tasks – gains more attention in the international discussion (Luthar, 2006; Wust-mann, 2004).

Research on resilience has identified several factors that strengthen the power and resources of children as well as promote their abilities to cope successfully with crises and internal and external problems: The most important protective factor is the stable, secure attachment to a significant adult, and its internal, intrapsychic representations. Luthar (2006, p. 780) summarizes the results of fifty years of resilience research as follows: The most important message is that resilience is fundamentally based on relationship and attachment.

A base for the establishment of a secure attachment is the positive regard of the child and an empathic, structured educational behaviour of parents/other adults. Further more, children need opportunities to built up a good self-esteem and a sense of self-efficacy and a fine support in the development of the ability to regulate one's emotions (self-regulation) (see Lösel, Bender, 2007; Luthar, 2006; Masten, 2001; Petermann et al., 2004; Walsh, 2003; Werner, 2007; Wust-mann, 2004).

Resilience is developing in the course of life, the early childhood years being of special importance. Resilience is a dynamic characteristic. Its development depends on experiences made whilst managing difficulties in real life, developmental tasks and overcoming crises. The successful coping or handling of these challenges has a positive effect on the power of resilience. Summing up the results of resilience research, six central factors which promote coping with developmental tasks, actual crisis and expectations can be distinguished (Bengel, Meinders-Lücking, Rottmann, 2009; Fröhlich-Gildhoff, Dörner, Rön-nau, 2012):

Also, the concept of resilience is similar to the concept of life skills (UNICEF, 2011; WHO, 1994, a comparison was made by Fröhlich-Gildhoff, Rönnau-Böse, 2011).

The Importance of Prevention

Current research results in developmental psychology, educational research, developmental sciences and (neurobiological) learning research (e.g., Dornes, 2000; Hüther, 2005; Petermann et al., 2004) impressively document the importance of early childhood years for the cognitive, emotional and social development of children. This leads to the necessity to promote the mental health's protective factors on a personal level in early years.

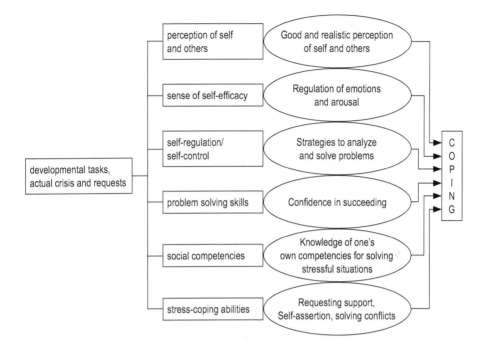

Figure 1. Six resilience factors

Meta-analysis of prevention studies show:

- Preventive programmes are more successful in a multi, systemic approach (reaching children and parents and professionals; setting-approach);
- Long-term programmes (> 6 months) are more successful than short-term projects or isolated trainings;
- Well structured programmes with behaviour-oriented strategies are more successful than "open" programmes;
- The promotion of general developmental abilities has better long-term effects than the prevention of isolated behavioural problems (e.g., aggressive behaviour) (summarized from Beelmann, 2006; Bengel et al., 2009; Durlak, Wells, 1997; Durlak, 2003; Heinrichs, Saßmann, Hahlweg, Perrez, 2002).

In several countries children are offered relatively complex programmes that focus on prevention for different target groups, for example 'high-risk-families', or focus on the promotion of special (part-) skills (like the stress-reduction programme of Klein-Heßling, Lohaus, 2000) or the prevention of specific behavioural disorders (e.g., the "Faustlos programme," Cierpka, 2005, for the prevention of violent behaviour). One problem is that most of the programmes are created (and evaluated) for school children. The other problem is that these programmes are often not involved in a setting approach, especially for early childhood institutions.

Early childhood institutions have a great influence on a child's development, because they are instances of central socialisation – they are often the first institutions where professionals are involved in education besides the family (e.g., Fthenakis, 2003; Kasüschke, Fröhlich-Gildhoff, 2008; Sylva, Melhuish, Sammons, Siraj-Blatchford, Taggart, Elliot, 2003). They address young children – and in modern form (e.g., Early Excellence Centres in the UK) the parents as well.

These institutions provide good opportunities for the implementation of prevention programmes in a setting approach. They are usually well-established and embedded in the local area and can easily identify the needs of children and their families. The early childhood teachers could have an elementary influence on the development of children as well as their families. The professionals must be prepared/trained for these (new) tasks and they need practicable guidance (handbook/manual, process descriptions, etc.) in order to act systematically. A prevention programme has to use the institutions' professional resources.

The promotion of resilience and the implementation of prevention programmes to foster mental health and emotional well-being, especially among young children is even more important in deprived areas as these are characterized, for example, by high unemployment and poverty rates, a high level of diversity, bad public infrastructure and so on. Research has shown that the socio-economic status of families has an alarmingly high impact on readiness for school and school achievement, due to differences in speech development, social skills, self-regulation-abilities, motivation, cognitive development and self-efficacy-experiences (e.g., Duncan, Brooks-Gunn, 1997; Smith, Brooks-Gunn, Klevanov, 1997; Bengel et al., 2009). For young children growing up in such adverse conditions, acquiring skills as early as possible to cope positively with those strains is imperative. There are also high correlations between the social status and mental health indicators: A low socio-economic status is a risk factor for mental disorders (e.g. Ravens-Sieberer et al., 2007; Bengel et al., 2009).

The Project "Prevention of Exclusion – Promotion of resilience and mental health in early childhood institutions in deprived areas"

The research project "Prevention of Exclusion" was based on these theoretical findings and aimed at realising a concept for the promotion of resilience for preschool children in disadvantaged areas and evaluating its effects. The project, which was financed by the German Ministry for Education and Research (BMBF 2008–2010), was conducted in three German regions (Südbaden, Frankfurt,

Berlin) in five kindergartens in areas with high levels of poverty among families (mostly with migrant background).

A programme that wants to promote sustainable resilience in children needs to consider the personal, social and environmental factors that influence the development of a child. All resources with positive effects had to be used in such a programme. Therefore, the concept of promoting resilience was preventative in nature and followed a 'setting approach' (WHO, 2011) focussing on four different levels:

**Course of action:
integrated concept**

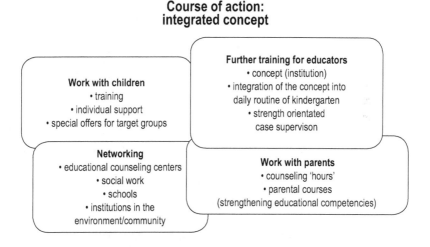

Figure 2. Integrated setting approach

Early childhood educators' level

The early childhood teachers in participating kindergartens (early childhood institutions) were involved in the work right from the beginning; this was necessary to ensure the sustainability of the project. Working on the educators' attitude formed the basis of the implementation of the concept for children and parents: the resource-orientated view, which refers to orientation of children's strengths, skills and self-competences, were fundamental to a holistic promotion of mental health and resilience. Here, relationships and attitudes which needed to be characterized by empathy, congruence and unconditional positive regard were of great importance. The realization of these variables aimed at helping children to build up a positive concept of self and to perceive themselves as an autonomous person (cf. Biermann-Ratjen, 2002).

During the two-year term of the project, the early childhood teachers received six further training sessions, covering topics such as the concept of resilience, methods for working with children and parents (resilience courses for children and parental courses – see subsequent method descriptions at child level and at parental level) and networking. Supervision meetings, where different "cases studies" were discussed from the perspective of promoting resilience, took place on a monthly basis.

Childrens' level

All children attending the institutions at the beginning of the project took part in a structured child-training-course, aimed at prevention as well as promotion of resilience (programme 'PRiK': Prevention and Resilience-promotion in Kindergarten, Fröhlich-Gildhoff et al., 2012). The theoretical basis of this course were the six protective factors (see above) which promote the resilience of children against stress and strains and improve their coping competences in crisis situations.

The children's course consisted of a ten-week-programme based on a training manual with six different modules. Each of the six modules comprised three or four units in which the topics were adequately modified for children. Altogether the children's course comprised twenty units. The concept of these modules was to help children gain positive experiences that are conducive to their further development. It was therefore fundamental that they underwent these experiences on their own (see Schmidtchen, 2001, p. 95). "Learning by making own experiences implicates personal engagement; the whole person with his or her feelings, as well as his or her cognitive aspects participates in the learning process" (Rogers, 1974, p. 13).

For example the first module, its topic being self-perception, was about getting to know oneself better on the one hand and on the other hand about integrating others' perception of oneself into one's concept of self. The child should become "aware of his or her own experiences and of him- or herself as an experiencing person and should develop a self-concept through these experiences" (Biermann-Ratjen, 2002, p. 16).

Parental level

Parents were given two offers during the project: A weekly family consultation hour was established where parents could take advantage of educational counselling on a non-committal basis. Parental courses were also established. The manual's structure and its various elements, comparable to relatively well evaluated programmes (cf., e.g., Heinrichs et al., 2002; Heinrichs, Krüger, Gruse, 2006), aimed at strengthening the parents in their parenting and relationship building skills (e.g., "Starke Eltern – Starke Kinder," Honkanen-Schoberth 2003; Tschöpe-Scheffler, 2003, 2006). The parental courses offered in the project (concept and evaluation data: Fröhlich-Gildhoff, Rönnau, Dörner, 2008) focused even more consistently on the parents' resources and provided links to the promotion of the children's resilience. A parental course comprised six units and took place once a week for one and a half hours. The courses were held in the early childhood institution, always attended by one of the early childhood educators. Participation was free of charge, which lowered the threshold for accessing the course. However, parents that were "difficult to reach" could only be reached when other parents who had already attended the course started talking positively about it. Motivated by their reports and helpful experiences, parents who normally would not make use of such an offer, dared to participate in a course.

Network level

Another element of the project was to develop the cooperation and networking between the early childhood institutions and other institutions. In a first step, network maps for each institution were drafted to describe the current situation: The kind of cooperation they had, the institutions that were involved and how the kindergarten was located in the area. During the project a close cooperation with the responsible educational guidance institutions was built which led to "short cuts" in the way families approached these institutions.

Evaluation

The project was evaluated in a complex design. The following research questions had to be answered:
- Is it possible to reach children and parents, living in high risk areas, through a multi-level approach carried out by the early childhood institutions and its professionals?
- Are there effects on the children's concept of self, especially self-esteem, their problem solving skills, their social-emotional skills and (perhaps) other developmental factors?
- Are there variations in the children's behaviour during the project and in the pre/post comparison?
- Are there changes in the attitudes and behaviour of the participating professionals (early childhood teachers)?
- In which way did the parents participate in the project and are there detectable effects on the parents' development?

To evaluate the complex programme a combination of process and outcome evaluation with quantitative and qualitative methods was chosen; the evaluation was realised in a control-group design (with intervention group IG and control group CG). There were three measuring points: At the beginning of the project (t0), after six months, when a proportion of children left the kindergarten ("kindergarten-kids," t1) and after eighteen months, at the end of the project (t2), see Figure 3.

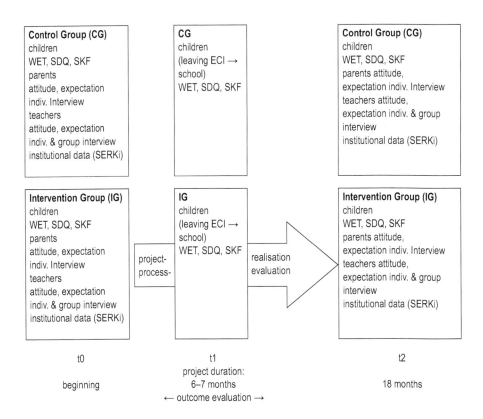

Figure 3. Evaluation design

Method

Participants

Five early childhood institutions participated in the Intervention Group (IG), with 349 children; in the Control Group (CG) five kindergartens also participated with 367 children. All early childhood institutions were located in areas with a high percentage of poor families. The quotient of families with immigrant background in the IG was between 100% and 28,1% (Mean 57,1%), and between 90.9% and 4.9% (Mean 60.6%) in the CG, χ^2 (1, $\underline{N}$ = 716) = 0,455, $\underline{p}$ = .486. There were no significant differences between the groups in the pre data in all quantitative instruments at t0.

Table 1 shows the number of participants and complete data versions at the different testing points. The return of complete data between t0 and t2 differs between 50.7% (data from parents) and 64.2% (data from the pedagogues); the children's data return is 62%. There was no difference in the contingent of missing data between CG and IG. The main reasons for the lost data were: relocation of families, change of professionals, illness of the young children at the testing points and lack of capacity to motivate the parents to fill out the questionnaires.

Table 1. Number of participants and complete data (in brackets: percentage of return of questionnaires)

	Children	Parents	Early childhood teachers	
Participating	$N = 716$ (349 IG, 367 CG)	$N = 515$	$N = 139$	
Testing t0 (complete data, all children)	$N = 424$	$N = 436$	$N = 564$	data reported about children by the teachers (SDQ)
t1 (only the children going to school)	$N = 150$	$N = 99$	$N = 179$	data reported about children by the teachers (SDQ)
Testing t2 (complete data, all children)	$N = 170$ (62%)	$N = 171$ (50.7%)	$N = 247$ (64.2%)	data reported about children by the teachers (SDQ)

Instruments

The evaluation instruments were selected according to the factors of resilience to be identified, i.e., they were chosen according to which methods would be most suitable for recording and documenting a development, especially changes in self-perception, self-efficacy, self-control, social competency, coping with stress and problem solving: The following quantitative instruments were chosen pre and post for both groups (Intervention Group IG and CG):

- Wiener Entwicklungstest (WET, Wiener development test; Kastner-Koller, Deimann, 2002) to measure the cognitive and social-emotional development of the children. The WET is a well advanced, standardized and normed instrument for measuring cognitive, linguistic and social-emotional development in a wide range.
- Selbstkonzeptfragebogen für Kinder im Vorschulalter (SKF, Self concept questionnaire for preschool children, Engel, Rönnau-Böse, Beuter, Wünsche, Fröhlich-Gildhoff, 2010) to measure the development in self-perception and self-concept of the children, The SKF is a standardized instrument (questionnaire) for measuring the concept of self in children aged 4–6 years by self report. The three scales anxiety/expectation of disappointment, physical (body) self concept and abilities show Cronbach-alpha data between $\alpha = .79$ und $\alpha = .83$.
- Strengths and Difficulties Questionnaire (SDQ, Goodman, 2005) to measure the development in children's behaviour. The SDQ is an internationally used, standardized and normed instrument (questionnaire); it is a brief behavioural screening questionnaire about 3–16 year olds. It exists in

126

several versions to meet the needs of researchers, clinicians and educators. The twenty five items (five scales: emotional symptoms, conduct problems, hyperactivity/inattention, peer relationship problems, and prosocial behaviour) are answered by teachers or parents.

The possible effects of the project on parents and early childhood teachers are covered by qualitative research methods. A possible change in attitudes and approaches could better be detected with qualitative methods than with questionnaires. For the qualitative evaluation, there were individual interviews (with parents and preschool teachers) conducted pre and post. The interpretation followed the principles of content analysis (e.g., Mayring, 2003[2]).

As an external evaluation, group interviews/discussions (e.g., Bohnsack, Nentwig-Gesemann, 2010) with the early childhood teachers were conducted pre and post in IG and CG, too (Nentwig-Gesemann, 2011; see Figure 4). The interpretation followed the principles of the "documentaric method" (Bohnsack, Nentwig-Gesemann, 2010).

Additionally all steps and elements of the process were documented in detail with standardised instruments, and records were kept during the project. They included children's training, parental courses, supervision, family consulting hours and conferences as well as reflection with the project leaders in their institutions.

Design of the external Evaluation

Group discussions (Bohnsack, Nentwig-Gesemann, 2010) with the pedagogues (early childhood teachers) (7 discussions in 7 teams) pre and post => N = 2 × 7 discussions with 75 pedagogues)

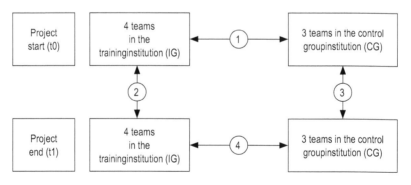

Comparison levels:
1 IG – CG at project's start   3 CG – CG pre/post
2 IG – IG pre/post   4 IG – CG at project's end

Figure 4. Design of the external evaluation

---

[2] In the content analysis, categories were defined from the empirical material (transcripts of the interviews). These categories were developed in an inductive and a deductive way (Mayring, 2003). The rating (classification of the empirical material) was assured in interrater workshops.

Results

In the following section, we will present a selection of the study's main results. A detailed description can be found in the final report (Fröhlich-Gildhoff, Beuter, Lindenberg, Rönnau-Böse, 2011).

The children's development

The people working in the project, the pedagogues/early childhood teachers, and the parents reported positive development among the children in the treatment-group. This could be identified by the process-documentation-instruments that were evaluated by means of content analysis by the pedagogues and parents.

The standardised instruments were analysed by statistical methods, especially multivariate variance analysis and further significance tests.

Development in cognitive and emotional skills. All in all, there was a development in the subtests of the WET (Wiener Entwicklungstest [Wiener development test], Kastner-Koller, Deimann, 2002) from t0 to t2:

Table 2. Results of variance analysis (time effects)

| | IG CG Effects of time | | | | | | |
	Pre M (SD)	Post M (SD)	Pre M (SD)	Post M (SD)	F	df	p
Schatzkästchen (treasure box)	4,35 (2,00)	4,59 (2,39)	5,09 (1,75)	5,09 (2,20)	0,365	155	.547
Zahlen Merken (remembering numbers)	4,84 (2,14)	4,92 (2,13)	4,34 (2,57)	5,48 (2,37)	9,789	152	**.002**
Gegensätze (contrasts)	3,01 (2,36)	4,36 (2,66)	3,27 (2,54)	4,58 (2,30)	66,669	153	**.000**
Bunte Formen (coloured forms)	4,42 (2,14)	5,58 (2,44)	5,10 (2,21)	5,53 (2,97)	8,875	116	**.004**
Quiz	3,21 (2,14)	3,43 (2,29)	3,10 (2,33)	4,38 (2,73)	14,663	138	**.000**
Fotoalbum (photo, measuring emotional development)	4,43 (2,13)	5,51 (2,30)	5,04 (2,24)	5,53 (2,39)	12,931	158	**.000**
Total Test-Score	4,04 (1,36)	4,75 (1,68)	4,28 (1,50)	4,91 (1,57)	34,615	163	**.000**

In the field of logical thinking (subtests "Quiz" and "Contrasts") and emotional development (subtest "Fotoalbum") the pre/post differences were significant. Even the total score of the WET showed a significant positive modification. Further statistic analysis showed significant developments (difference pre – post) in the IG, but not in the CG in the subtests Fotoalbum (measuring emotional development), IG: $\underline{t}$ (81) = 3.764, $\underline{p}$ < .001, $\underline{d}$ = 0.49; CG: $\underline{t}$ (77) = 1.457, $\underline{p}$ = .144, $\underline{d}$ = 0,21)] and "Bunte Formen" (measuring inductive thinking), IG: $\underline{t}$ (58) = 3.079, $\underline{p}$ = .003; $\underline{d}$ = 0.51; CG: $\underline{t}$ (58) = 1.133, $\underline{p}$ = .262; $\underline{d}$ = 0.17].

Development of the concept of self. At child level, the self-concept questionnaire (SKF; Engel et al., 2010) was applied. The results showed a significant positive development in the scale anxiety/expectation of disappointment in the IG, but not in the CG. This means that the children who took part in the project developed better self-confidence and stronger self-esteem (see Table 3). The effects in the variance analysis were proven by post hoc significance tests. These showed a significant positive development only in the IG.

Table 3. Scale anxiety/expectation of disappointment – post hoc tests (Higher scores mean lower anxiety)

	t(0)	t(2)				t(0)	t(2)			
			IG		**t-Test**			**CG**		**t-Test**
			$\underline{t}$	$\underline{df}$	$\underline{p}$			$\underline{t}$	$\underline{df}$	p
	$\underline{M}$ (SD)	$\underline{M}$ (SD)					$\underline{M}$ (SD)	$\underline{M}$ (SD)			
anxiety/ expectation of disappointment	25,79 (6,61)	29,27 (5,17)	3,540	55	**.001**	28,21 (5,55)	29,36 (5,88)	1,200	55	.235

Table 4. Means, standard deviation and results of the variance analysis of the Strength and Difficulties Questionnaires, IG and CG

IG	IG		Time effects		
	Pre	Post	t	df	p
	$\underline{M}$ (SD)	$\underline{M}$ (SD)			
Emotional Problems	2,05 (1,89)	2,88 (6,87)	1,108	85	.271
Externalising Behaviour Problems	2,52 (1,79)	1,79 (1,63)	3,369	84	**.001**
Hyperactivity	3,39 (2,41)	3,56 (2,48)	0,771	83	.443
Problems with peers	2,12 (1,75)	1,73 (1,59)	2,058	83	**.043**
Prosocial behaviour	7,69 (1,69)	8,27 (1,65)	2,820	82	**.006**
CG					
Emotional Problems	1,75 (1,60)	1,84 (1,99)	0,297	43	.768
Externalising Behaviour Problems	2,28 (1,53)	1,80 (1,63)	2,139	45	**.038**
Hyperactivity	4,19 (2,55)	3,81 (2,22)	1,597	42	.118
Problems with peers	1,64 (1,59)	1,49 (1,59)	0,673	44	.505
Prosocial behaviour	7,82 (1,54)	7,82 (1,70)	0,000	43	.999

Development of behavior. The analysis of the Strengths and Difficulties Questionnaire (Goodman, 2005) showed in the parents' version that the parents of the IG assessed significant changes in the scales behaviour problems (decreasing), social problems with peers (decreasing), and prosocial behaviour (increasing; see Table 4). In the CG there was only a comparable change in the scale behaviour problems.

Interviews with educators and parents (mostly mothers) revealed that they recognised changes in the behaviour of their children due to the project. For example, some of the children showed:

- Application of simple practical methods in everyday life in kindergarten, e.g., children using the 'emotion clock' to express their mood (The 'emotion clock' shows several faces which express different states of mood. By means of a clock's hands the children can show their feelings).
- More independence and self-confidence.
- Advanced ability to communicate feelings and limits.

Development of the early childhood teachers

Compared to the situation at the beginning of the project, cooperation within the teams of the early childhood institutions improved. The concept of the trainings was to give new impetus to the subject of resilience, to provide a forum to exchange opinions with colleagues as well as to provide an opportunity to reflect on typical work days. In the qualitative evaluation most of the preschool teachers of the IG (68% identified in the pre/post group discussions) showed changes in their attitudes: they more often recognised the children's resources and strengths and they had more empathy with individuals.

Cooperation with parents improved (results of the analysis of the process documentation). Professionals could focus on families' specific situations and could give them more tailored support (e.g., in questions concerning educational skills development). In most of the teams the atmosphere improved, grew more positive. The pedagogues discovered the extent of their own competencies and the teams' resources and competencies; they reported for example, an increase in skills for purposes of communication and child-orientated interventions (results of the group discussions and the single interviews).

The professionals in the kindergartens in the disadvantaged quarters felt a greater emotional burden, and needed specific support to protect their own mental health (interview data).

Development of parents

The parents felt supported by the training courses and the individual counselling sessions (results from the analysis of the qualitative data/interviews). Course attendance was approximately 47%, while another group of parents (29%)

benefited from individual counselling, which also made the access to these parents easier.

Parents in the interviews described how they were now more capable of recognising their own competencies and that they felt more confident in educational tasks in daily situations – this was a new experience for them. In comparison with the control-group the parents from the institutions involved felt more secure in their educational competencies at the end of the project.

Discussion

The project showed in general, that it was possible to implement a strategy for the promotion of mental health, oriented at specific resilience factors, in a multimodal setting approach in early childhood institutions in disadvantaged areas. The professionals – early childhood teachers – could be involved systematically in the preventive programme; they were enabled to implement measures to strengthen the children's resources and resilience-competencies. They developed their competencies in the cooperation with the families as well and continued the programme independently. This strategy leads to sustainability beyond the project's duration.

In addition to the previous project (Rönnau et al., 2008), the instruments and methods needed to be adapted to the specific situation of the families, and there was a need for more practical methods.

The project's integrated, multimodal intervention approach was evaluated by an combination of quantitative and qualitative methods. The evaluation showed positive results on a qualitative and quantitative level; these results are in line with the results of other studies, i.e., Lösel Beelmann, Stemmler, and Jaursch (2006, see also Beelmann, Lösel, 2004). In detail, the results of the children (in the intervention group) showed – compared with the control-group and over time – a couple of positive changes, especially concerning the development of self-esteem. Positive effects were also seen in the children's behaviour (especially assessed by their parents).

The positive effects in cognitive developmental factors – measured with the quantitative instruments – were not so distinct as they were in the previous project (Rönnau et al., 2008). One reason might be, that the development of the children (and their parents) in the disadvantaged situations is 'slower' and needs more resources. Nevertheless, the project showed a lot of ways, possibilities and methods to reach the specific target group and to involve them in this systematic project. Another reason was that the quantitative instrument WET was not adapted to the specific situation, especially language problems, of children with migrant background. There exists a lack of evaluation-instruments for this group of children: The instruments were a challenge for the children and the parents of the specific target groups, for some of them the phrasing or style of the items was hard to understand. There is a desideratum for culture-adapted research instruments (other research teams had similar experiences, e.g., Fuhrer, Uslucan, 2005; Leyendecker, 2003).

The project showed – beside the measurable results – some important general experiences that promote the development of children:

- The early childhood institutions have the opportunity of reaching the parents in a successful way, to contact and to motivate them to cooperate. For example, parents can be addressed when bringing and picking up their children. A high degree of transparency in all steps of the intervention has had a positive effect on the parents' motivation.
- The parents appreciate the combination of group offers (parental courses) and the possibility of one-to-one consultation – those parents who did not attend the parental courses could be addressed in the counselling sessions. This illustrates the necessity of a diverse range of services in order to reach as many parents (groups) as possible and confirms likewise the results of other studies (BMFSFJ/DJI, 2006; Fröhlich-Gildhoff, Kraus-Gruner, Rönnau, 2006).
- Close co-operation between the early childhood institutions and the educational guidance institutions had a positive effect. The early childhood teachers felt well supported and for the parents it became easier to get in contact with the educational guidance.
- A change in the perspective regarding the resources and strengths of the children had the effect that both educators and parents had a more positive perception of the children and of their own skills. This led to a more relaxed atmosphere, other courses of action and increased confidence on both sides.

Research in developmental psychology (e.g., Stern, 1992), psychotherapy (e.g., Grawe, 2004; Norcross, 2002) and resilience (Luthar, 2006) confirmed the central influence of the relationship between (professional) adults and children on children's mental health. In the last years, Pianta and colleagues (Pianta, Stuhlman, Hamre, 2007) gave hints regarding which key roles professional staff can play in early childhood institutions and schools for the children's development – provided that they meet the children's needs and attachment-styles. Then the children can create new experiences, reflect on these experiences and integrate them into their self-image. These effects were supported by the qualitative results of the project: The trainers in the children's and in the parental courses were questioned about their authenticity, their sensibility and their empathy. The course programmes and its manuals had been a frame for the processes in the children's and parental groups. It gave some kind of structure, but the person-to-person interaction between the trainer and the group members (and among the group members) had a stronger impact. This was shown in the behaviour of the children during the group-sessions (proved by the records) and by the data of the parents' interviews.

All in all, the results show a good opportunity for early childhood institutions in high-risk areas and their professionals to reach young children (and their parents) to promote resilience and to strengthen coping abilities. In this way the prevention programme can boost protective factors and avoid developmental problems later on. The project's findings document the necessity of a multilevel approach to promote mental health and social emotional wellbeing of children by the professionals in early childhood institutions – this knowledge should be a relevant part of educational strategies and professional training, too.

Outlook

Due to the positive results the concept of resilience promotion was adapted to the situation of primary schools (Becker, 2012; Fröhlich-Gildhoff, Becker, Fischer, 2012). In Germany a new project started ("Grundschule macht stark;" primary school strengthen children) with ten primary schools. A Systematic and coordinated intervention is realized on four levels.

School level: Organisational development (vision, concept, tasks)

Teacher level: qualification/competence development: strengthening the social and emotional wellbeing of children; qualification to realize resilience promoting courses in the classes (concept: Fröhlich-Gildhoff, Becker, Fischer, 2012).

Class/group level: Pupils: specific interventions (courses) for the promotion of resilience.

Parents: interventions/measures to strengthen educational competencies.

Individual level: specific support for children and parents in crisis/risky situations.

First experiences show, that it needs more time to reflect primary school teachers' attitudes. Mostly they understand themselves more as subject teacher for mathematics, language etc. and less as pedagogues with the task of strengthening pupils' socio-emotional competences. But nevertheless it is possible to change the professionals' views and to move to resilience focused interventions.

References

Beelmann, A. (2006). Wirksamkeit von Präventionsmaßnahmen bei Kindern und Jugendlichen: Ergebnisse und Implikationen der integrativen Erfolgsforschung [Effectivenes of prevention measures with children and adolsecents: Results and implications of integrative outcome research]. *Zeitschrift für klinische Psychologie und Psychotherapie*, 35(2), 151–162.

Beelmann, A., Lösel, F. (2004). *Elterntraining zur Förderung der Erziehungskompetenz* [Parental training]. München, Germany: Juventa.

Bengel, J., Meinders-Lücking, F., Rottmann, N. (2009). *Schutzfaktoren bei Kindern und Jugendlichen. Stand der Forschung zu psychosozialen Schutzfaktoren für Gesundheit. Forschung und Praxis der Gesundheitsförderung* 35 [Protecting factors review about research]. Köln, Germany: BZgA.

Biermann-Ratjen, E.-M. (2002). *Entwicklungspsychologie und Störungslehre* [Developmental psychology and theory of disorders]. [In:] C. Boeck-Singelmann, B. Ehler, T. Hensel, F. Kemper, C. Monden-Engelhardt (Eds.). *Personzentrierte Psychotherapie mit Kindern und Jugendlichen* (Vol. 1, 11–34). Göttingen, Germany: Hogrefe.

Bohnsack, R., Nentwig-Gesemann, I. (Eds.). (2010). *Dokumentarische Evaluationsforschung. Theoretische Grundlagen und Beispiele aus der Praxis* [Documentaric evaluation methods]. Opladen, Germany: B. Budrich.

Bundesministerium für Familie, Frauen, Senioren und Jugend (BMFSFJ)/Deutsches Jugendinstitut (DJI) (2006). *Kurzevaluation von Programmen zu Frühen Hilfen für Eltern und Kinder und sozialen Frühwarnsystemen in den Bundesländern* [Short evaluation on early support for families and children]. Abschlussbericht. Berlin, Germany: Eigendruck des BMFSFJ; auch zu beziehen über www.bmfsfj.de.

Cicchetti, D., Cohen, D.J. (Eds.). (2006). *Developmental Psychopathology: Risk, disorder, and adaptation* (2nd ed.). New York: Wiley.

Cierpka, M. (2005). *FAUSTLOS – Wie Kinder Konflikte gewaltfrei lösen lernen* [FAUSTLOS – a programme for the prevention of aggressive behaviour]. Freiburg, Germany: Herder.

Dornes, M. (2000). *Die emotionale Welt des Kindes* [The emotional world of the child]. Frankfurt a.M., Germany: Fischer.

Duncan, G.J., Brooks-Gunn, J. (1997). *Consequences of growing up poor*. New York: Russell Sage Press.

Durlak, J.A. (2003). Generalizations regarding effective prevention and health promotion programs. [In:] T.P. Gullotta, M. Bloom (Eds.). *The encyclopedia of primary prevention and health promotion* (61—69). New York: Kluwer Academic/Plenum.

Durlak, J.A., Wells, A.M. (1997). Primary prevention mental health programs for children and adolescents. A meta-analytic review. *American Journal of Community Psychology*, 25, 115—152.

Engel, E.-M., Rönnau-Böse, M., Beuter, S., Wünsche, M., Fröhlich-Gildhoff, K. (2010). *Selbstkonzeptfragebogen für Kinder im Vorschulalter (SKF) – Konzept, Entwicklung und praktische Erfahrungen* [Self concept questionnaire for preschool children]. [In:] K. Fröhlich-Gildhoff, I. Nentwig-Gesemann, P. Strehmel (Eds.). *Forschung in der Frühpädagogik III. Schwerpunkt Sprachentwicklung und Sprachförderung* (305–328). Freiburg, Germany: FEL.

Fröhlich-Gildhoff, K., Becker, J., Fischer, S. (2012). *Prävention und Resilienzförderung in Grundschulen (PRiGS). Ein Förderprogramm.* [Prevention and promotion of resilience in primary schools]. München: Reinhardt.

Fröhlich-Gildhoff, K., Dörner, T., Rönnau, M. (2012). *PRiK – Prävention und Resilienzförderung in Kindertagesstätten. Ein Trainingsprogramm* [Prevention and pomotion of resilience in kindergarten – a trainings programme] (2nd ed.). München, Germany: Reinhardt.

Fröhlich-Gildhoff, K., Rönnau-Böse, M. (2012a). Prevention of exclusion: the promotion of resilience in early childhood institutions in disadvantaged areas. *Journal of Public Health*: Vol. 20, Issue 2 (2012), 131–139.

Fröhlich-Gildhoff, K., Rönnau-Böse, M. (2012). The Promotion of Mental Health in Early Childhood Institutions (ECI) under a Person-Centred Perspective. *Hellenic Journal of Psychology*, Vol. 9(2012), 255–277.

Fröhlich-Gildhoff, K., Beuter, S., Lindenberg, J., Rönnau-Böse, M. (2011). *Förderung der seelischen Gesundheit in Kitas bei Kindern und Familien mit sozialen Benachteiligungen* [Promotion of mental health in early childhood institutions in deprived areas]. [Abschlussbericht des Projekts „Prävention zur Verhinderung von Exklusion. Förderung der seelischen Gesundheit in Einrichtungen der Kindertagesbetreuung in Quartieren mit besonderen Problemlagen"]. Freiburg, Germany: FEL.

Fröhlich-Gildhoff, K., Rönnau-Böse, M. (2011). *Resilienz* [Resilience] (2nd ed.). München, Germany: Reinhardt/UTB.

Fröhlich-Gildhoff, K. (2008). *Effective factors in child and adolescent therapy*. [In:] M. Behr, J. Cornelius-White (Eds.). *Facilitating young people's development. International perspectives on person-centred theory and practice* (25–39). Ross-on-Wye, UK: PCCS Books

Fröhlich-Gildhoff, K., Rönnau, M., Dörner, T. (2008). *Eltern stärken mit Kursen in Kitas* [Strengthening parents with courses in kindergarten]. München, Germany: Reinhardt.

Fröhlich-Gildhoff, K., Kraus-Gruner, G., Rönnau, M. (2006). Gemeinsam auf dem Weg. Eltern und Erzieher Innen gestalten Erziehungspartnerschaft [Partnership between parents and early childhood teachers]. *Kindergarten heute*, 10, 6–15.

Fthenakis, W.E. (Eds.). (2003). *Elementarpädagogik nach PISA. Wie aus Kindertagesstätten Bildungseinrichtungen werden können* [Early childhood education beyond PISA. The development of kindergarten to educaional institutions]. Freiburg, Germany: Herder.

Fuhrer, U., Uslucan, H.-H. (Eds.). (2005). *Familie, Akkulturation und Erziehung. Migration zwischen Eigen- und Fremdkultur* [Family, acculturation and education. Migration between cultures]. Stuttgart, Germany: Kohlhammer.

Gendlin, G. (1981). *Focusing. Technik der Selbsthilfe bei der Lösung persönlicher Probleme* [Focusing. Techniques of self support by personal problems]. Salzburg, Austria: Müller.

Goodman, R. (2005). Strengths and Difficulties Questionnaire. Retrieved March 4, 2011, from http://www.sdqinfo.org/py/doc/b3.py?language = German.

Goodman, R. (2001). Psychometric properties of the Strengths and Difficulties Questionnaire (SDQ). *Journal of the American Academy of Child and Adolescent Psychiatry*, 40, 1337–1345.

Grawe, K. (2004). *Neuropsychotherapie.* [Neuropsychotherapy] Göttingen, Germany: Hogrefe.

Grawe, K., Donati, R., Bernauer, F. (1994). *Psychotherapie im Wandel. Von der Konfession zur Profession* [Psychotherapy in change. From confession to profession]. Göttingen, Germany: Hogrefe.

Heinrichs, N., Saßmann, H., Hahlweg, K., Perrez, M. (2002). Prävention kindlicher Verhaltensstörungen [Prevention of behavioural disorders]. *Psychologische Rundschau*, 53, 170–183.

Heinrichs, N., Krüger, S., Gruse, U. (2006). Der Einfluss von Anreizen auf die Rekrutierung von Eltern und auf die Effektivität eines präventiven Elterntrainings

[The influence of incentives on the efficacy of parental trainings]. *Zeitschrift für klinische Psychologie und Psychotherapie*, 35, 97–108.

Honkanen-Schoberth, P. (2003). *Starke Kinder brauchen starke Eltern. Der Elternkurs des Deutschen Kinderschutzbundes* [Strong children need strong parents. A parental course] (2nd ed.). Berlin, Germany: Eigendruck Deutscher Kinderschutzbund. see also: http://www.elternkurs-schulung.de.

Hüther, G. (2005). *Die Macht der inneren Bilder. Wie Visionen das Gehirn den Menschen und die Welt verändern* [The power of internal pictures. How visions could change neuronal structures]. Göttingen, Germany: Vandenhoeck and Rupprecht.

Kastner-Koller, U., Deimann, P. (2002). *Wiener Entwicklungstest* [Wiener developmental test]. Göttingen, Germany: Hogrefe.

Kasüschke, D., Fröhlich-Gildhoff, K. (2008). *Frühpädagogik heute* [Early childhood education today]. Köln, Germany: WoltersKluwer.

Klein-Heßling, J., Lohaus, A. (2000). *Streßpräventionstraining für Kinder im Grundschulalter* [Stress prevention training for primary school kids] (2nd ed.). Göttingen, Germany: Hogrefe.

Leyendecker, B. (2003*).* Die frühe Kindheit in Migrantenfamilien. [In:] H. Keller (Ed.). *Handbuch der Kleinkindforschung [Early childhood in migrant families]* (3rd. ed., 381–432). Bern, Switzerland: Huber.

Lösel, F., Bender, D. (2007). *Von generellen Schutzfaktoren zu spezifischen protektiven Prozessen: Konzeptuelle Grundlagen und Ergebnisse der Resilienzforschung* [From general protective factors to specific protective processes. Basics and outcomes of resilience research]. [In:] G. Opp, M. Fingerle, A. Freytag (Eds.). *Was Kinder stärkt: Erziehung zwischen Risiko und Resilienz* (2nd ed., 57–78). München: Reinhardt.

Lösel, F., Beelmann, A., Stemmler, M., Jaursch, S. (2006). Prävention von Problemen des Sozialverhaltens im Vorschulalter: Evaluation des Eltern- und Kindertrainings EFFEKT [Prevention of problems in social behaviour in early childhood. Evaluation of the children and the parental training EFFEKT]. *Zeitschrift für Klinische Psychologie und Psychotherapie*, 35, 117–126.

Luthar, S.S. (2006). *Resilience in development: A synthesis of research across five decades.* [In:] D. Cicchetti, D.J. Cohen (Eds.). *Developmental Psychopathology: Risk, disorder, and adaptation* (2nd ed., 739–795). New York: Wiley.

Luthar, S.S., Cicchetti, D. (2000). The construct of resilience: Implications for interventions and social policies. *Development and Psychopathology*, 12, 857–885.

Masten, A.S. (2001). Ordinary magic: Resilience processes in development. *American Psychologist*, 56(3), 227–238.

Mayring, P. (2003). *Qualitative Inhaltsanalyse. Grundlagen und Techniken* [Qualitative content analysis. Basics and techniques]. Weinheim, Germany: Beltz.

Nentwig-Gesemann, I. (2011). *Ergebnisse der externen Evaluation des Projekts „Prävention zur Verhinderung von Exklusion. Förderung der seelischen Gesundheit in Einrichtungen der Kindertagesbetreuung in Quartieren mit besonderen Problemlagen"* [Results of the external evaluation of the project "Promotion of mental health in early childhood institutions in deprived areas"]. [In:] K. Fröhlich-Gildhoff, S. Beuter, J. Lindenberg, M. Rönnau-Böse (Eds.). *Förderung der seelischen Gesundheit in Kitas bei Kindern und Familien mit sozialen Benachteiligungen*, (135–152). Freiburg, Germany: FEL.

Norcross, J.C. (Ed.). (2002). *Psychotherapy relationships that work: Therapist contributions and responsiveness to patients*. Oxford: Universitiy Press.

Opp, G., Fingerle, M. (Eds.). (2007). *Was Kinder stärkt: Erziehung zwischen Risiko und Resilienz* [Strengthening children: education between risk and resilience] (2nd ed.). München, Germany: Reinhardt.

Petermann, F., Niebank, K., Scheithauer, H. (2004). *Entwicklungswissenschaft. Entwicklungspsychologie – Genetik – Neuropsychologie* [Developmental sciences. Developmental psychology – genetic – neuropsychology]. Berlin, Germany: Springer.

Pianta, R.C., Stuhlman, M.W., Hamre, B.K. (2007). *Der Einfluss von Erwachsenen-Kind-Beziehungen auf Resilienzprozesse im Vorschulalter und in der Grundschule* [The influence of adult-child-relationships on resilience processes of preschool in primary school children]. [In:] G. Opp, M. Fingerle (Eds.). *Was Kinder stärkt: Erziehung zwischen Risiko und Resilienz* (2nd ed., 192–211). München, Germany: Reinhardt.

Rönnau, M., Kraus-Gruner, G., Engel, E.-M. (2008). *Resilienzförderung in der Kindertagesstätte* [The promotion of resilience in early childhood institutions]. [In:] K. Fröhlich-Gildhoff, I. Nentwig-Gesemann, R. Haderlein (Eds.). *Forschung in der Frühpädagogik* (117–147). Freiburg, Germany: FEL.

Rogers, C.R. (1974). *Lernen in Freiheit* [Learning in freedom]. München, Germany: Kösel.

Schmidtchen, S. (2001). *Allgemeine Psychotherapie für Kinder, Jugendliche und Familien* [General psychotherapy for children and adolescents and families]. Stuttgart, Germany: Kohlhammer.

Smith, J.R., Brooks-Gunn, J., Klevanov, P.K. (1997). *Consequences of living in poverty for young children's cognitive and verbal ability and early school achievement.* [In:] G.J. Duncan, J. Brooks-Gunn (Eds.). *Consequences of growing up poor* (132–189). New York: Russell Sage Press.

Stern, D.N. (1992). *Die Lebenserfahrung des Säuglings.* Stuttgart: Klett-Cotta.

Sylva, K., Melhuish, E., Sammons, P., Siraj-Blatchford, I., Taggart, B., Elliot, K. (2003). *The effective provision of pre-school education (EPPE) project: Findings from the pre-school period.* London: University of London, Institute of Education.

Tschöpe-Scheffler, S. (2003). *Elternkurse auf dem Prüfstand. Wie Erziehung wieder Freude macht* [A Check of parental courses]. Opladen, Germany: Leske und Brudrich.

Tschöpe-Scheffler, S. (2006). *Konzepte der Elternbildung – Eine kritische Übersicht* [Concepts of parental education a critical review]. Opladen, Germany: Leske und Budrich.

UNICEF (2011). *Which skills are life skills?* Retrieved June 16, 2011, from http://www.unicef.org/lifeskills/index_whichskills.html (accessed 19.09.2012).

Walsh, F. (2003). Familiy resilience: Strengths forged through adversity. [In:] F. Walsh (Ed.). *Normal familiy processes: Growing diversity and complexity.* New York: Guilford.

Weinberger, S. (2001). *Kinder spielend helfen* [Play therapy]. Weinheim, Germany: Beltz.

Werner, E.E. (2007). *Resilienz. Ein Überblick über internationale Längsschnittstudien* [Resilience. An overview about international longitudinal studies]. [In:] G. Opp, M. Fingerle (Eds.). Was Kinder stärkt. Erziehung zwischen Risiko und Resilienz (2nd ed., 20–31). München, Germany: Ernst Reinhardt.

Werner, E.E. (1997). The value of applied research for Head Start: A cross-cultural and longitudinal Perspective. National Head Start Association. *Journal of Research and Evaluation,* 1, 15–24.

WHO (World Health Organisation) (2011). *Health settings.* Retrieved June 14, 2011, from http://www.who.int/healthy_settings/en.

WHO (World Health Organisation) (Ed.). (1994). *Life Skills Education in schools*. Genf, Switzerland: WHO.

Wustmann, C. (2004). *Resilienz. Widerstandsfähigkeit von Kindern in Tageseinrichtungen fördern* [Resilience. Promotion of children's ressources in early childhood institutions]. Weinheim, Germany: Beltz.

III. RESILIENCE AND DISEASE

Władysława Pilecka
Jagiellonian University
Institute of Psychology

RESILIENCE AS A CHANCE
OF DEVELOPMENTAL SUCCESS FOR A CHILD
WITH A CHRONIC ILLNESS

Abstract

Chronic physical illness considered as a negative event, a potential stressor or a life crisis can be the risk factor for difficulties in the development of a child. Negative consequences of transactional influence of the factors associated with illness parameters, a child's personality and his or her environment occur particularly in the emotional and social development. This situation can be also the chance for stimulating a development of a child's personality and his or her growing as a person. The theoretical construct that in right way explains the positive transformation in understanding of the context of chronic illness – is a resilience. The meaning of this construct is discussed from the perspective of model proposed by E. Groetberg and assumptions of positive psychology, while its application value is showed in the light of the empirical data. The conceptualization of a developmental success refers to psychological well-being and being a mature and optimally functioning person.

Key words: child with a chronic illness, resilience, developmental success, psychological well-being, mature and optimally functioning person

Chronic somatic diseases are a civilizational hallmark of the life of contemporary man at all stages of his development. Medical statistics of the last a few decade shave shown an increase in the incidence of some chronic conditions, e.g. diabetes type I, allergy, asthma, or cancers. It is assumed that about 31% of children and youth under 18 suffer from different somatic diseases more often characterized by a mild course (66%) than a moderate (29%) or severe one (5%), significantly limiting their everyday life activity (Newacheck, Taylor, 1992).

The contemporary understanding of a chronic somatic disease is based on the biopsychological model of health and disease perceiving disease as a potential stressor that transforms the life of the child and his or her family, entailing certain demands and limitations that the child and the family have to face up to. The process of coping with a new, difficult situation is called adaptation. It does not consist in passively adjusting to new requirements through behavior modifications but in a creative response to encountered difficulties and dangers, supposedly resulting in the end in a positive cost-benefit analysis. Somatic problems in children and youth are always connected with their social and emotional functioning that is either a cause or effect of such problems (Thompson, Gustafson, 1996; Pilecka 2002).

Contemporary research provides evidence that most children with chronic illnesses function as well as their healthy peers or in some cases even better (Barakat, Pulgaron, Daniel, 2009). R.B. Noll and M.J. Kapust (2007) believe that the so called *hardiness* is a theoretic construct that effectively explains why and in what way children diagnosed to suffer from cancer reach a successful level of psychosocial adaptation. At present, however, pediatric psychological literature far more often refers to the term *resilience* whose definitions strongly highlight factors constituting direct indicators of an effective adaptation to stressful circumstances.

How to understand resilience

psychological literature provides many definitions of resilience, all of them provoking critical discussions, highlighting the complexity and ambiguity of the term. Yet, as popularly understood, the concept seems easy to define. In the evolution of views on the essence of children's resilience, M. O'Dougherty-Wright and A. Masten (2006) distinguish three waves:
- wave I: identifying individual resilience and its determinants;
- wave II: embedding resilience in developmental and ecological systems, with a focus on its processes;
- wave III: fostering resilience through preventive interventions modifying the child's development.

At the time of the first wave, i.e. the latter half of the 70s and the first half of the 80s, researchers tried to accurately describe resilience, taking into account its different characteristics. Most often it was discussed with regard to positive adaptation to past and present adversities, with an assumption that resilience is responsible either for a general or unique level of this adaptation. As O'Dougherty-Wright and Masten state, researchers attempted to describe the criteria for resilience, and its internal and external determinants. Resilience was defined in the first place in terms of assets, compensatory or promoting factors enabling the child to achieve effective adaptation in all difficult situations, even those related to a highest risk. Resilience was attributed with particular

significance by some authors; they perceived it as a protective factor manifesting itself exclusively in high-risk situations. The determinants were usually divided into four groups:
- characteristics of the child: temperament qualities, good level of intellectual development, effective coping strategies, positive self-perception (self-confidence, high self-esteem, sense of self-effectiveness), positive attitude to life (attitude of hope), sense of meaning in life, traits important from the perspective of society (talents, sense of humor, attractiveness to others);
- characteristics of the family: stable and supporting home (rare conflicts, emotional closeness, parents' authority, positive relationships between siblings, support from more distant relatives), supporting the child in education, socioeconomic status, level of parent's education, religious beliefs;
- characteristics of the environment: good neighborly relations, education services, employment chances for parents and relatives, good healthcare, public safety services, significant persons and socially-minded peers;
- characteristics of the culture and social policy: legal protection of children, values promoted in education, prevention of and protection from political violence, low tolerance for physical violence.

During the second wave, particularly in the 90s, researchers endeavored to understand the processes leading to acquiring resilience in the course of human development. With that in mind, they drew on the achievements of biology, sociology and humanities in order to show relations the individual has with other systems at various levels of their organization during the whole life, and mechanisms that the individual uses to develop his or her own complex of adaptive mechanisms. The child's relations with his or her ecosystem context became a subject of the empirical studies of the time. The child's perception and interpretation of his or her experiences was acknowledged as a factor considerably modifying these relations. The significance that the child ascribes to these experiences determines the effect the context has on his or her adaptation and resilience. The very resilience was also described then as a dynamic and multidimensional process determined by transactional relations between individual and contextual factors. At that time, studies provided evidence that the same child can be diagnosed as resilient at a certain time of his or her life and not resilient at another one, that the child can show resilience in certain situations, and not in other ones; and finally, that the child can be resilient only to certain events in his or her life.

The third wave – the last decades – is characterized by an intense search for intentional ways of fostering resilience in children from risk groups and in children whose development is not disturbed. Basing on various theoretical assumptions, researchers started to construct programs intended to reinforce both individual and environmental assets of the child, and to reduce risk factors. Those programs are built with an intention to modify the behavior of parents, teachers, professionals, as well as children themselves. The programs can be of promoting or preventive, and of corrective, i.e. remedial, character.

Summing up the presented discussion it can be stated that in the subject literature resilience is most often defined descriptively at a varying level of generality. *Resilience is predominantly defined as children's ability, quality or competence to carry out their developmental tasks effectively or to achieve positive adaptation despite chronic problems, often severe ones, that they can face in the course of their life.*

The definition worked out by E. Grotberg (2000, p. 14), that is a definition of a high level of generality, says that resilience is a universal capacity which allows a person, group or community to prevent, minimize or overcome the damaging effects of adversity.

P. Wyman, I. Sandler, S. Wolchik and K. Nelson (2000, p. 133) believe on the other hand that resilience is a competence enabling the child to achieve positive developmental goals and avoid non-adaptive behaviors, particularly in crisis situations.

Another general definition is also the one proposed by M. Tyszkowa (1986). According to her resilience is an ability of an individual to oppose frustrating and stressing effects of a difficult situation by staying at a proper level of cognitive understanding of the situation and emotional control based on this understanding (p. 337).

Narrow-range definitions show resilience as a capacity to achieve positive goals by children from risk groups, i.e. those exposed to violence, poverty, permanent limitations or health-related risks, etc., a competence making it possible to effectively cope with stress or an ability to constructively struggle with trauma. In these definitions, resilience is perceived as one of personality dimensions, along with self-evaluation, locus of control, hardiness or temperament (quoted after: Jordan, 2006).

The role of resilience in the psychosocial development and functioning of children with chronic somatic diseases can be better understood in view of E. Grotberg's model and the theoretical assumptions of positive psychology.

Resilience according to Edith Grotberg

Among the factors highly determining resilience in childhood and adolescence are cognitive processes understood both as general intelligence as well as processing and organizing information about oneself in certain mental structures. General cognitive abilities constitute a strong and constant predicator of resilience. Children able to effectively solve cognitive problems will certainly manage well in difficult situations as they will have a richer and more diverse range of remedial strategies at hand. Apart from intelligence also abilities and skills of social cognition, i.e. factors responsible for the integration and safety of the I and for a sense of control, play here an important role. The most important cognitive patterns include: (1) the perception and evaluation of social support, (2) self-esteem, and (3) self-efficacy. The first pattern refers to the child's faith and trust in people around: the child believes that he or she is loved and can always count on being helped in difficult situations. The second oneis shaped on the basis of other people's opinions. The third pattern refers to the conviction that the set goals can be reached in spite of potential obstacles. High self-esteem and self-efficacy successfully protect the child against the negative effects of various risk factors.

E. Grotberg (2000) writes that there are three sources of resilience of the child: **I have**, **I am**, and **I can**. Factors within category **I have** include internal sources of support; according to the author, these are:

- interpersonal relationships based on trust: children at any age need both the unconditional love from their parents and caregivers, and positive emotions from other adults that can sometimes compensate the former ones;
- clear house rules: house rules and routines set tasks for the child who is rewarded for performing them, and, consequently, should accept them more easily; when the child does not follow the accepted rules, he or she is helped to understand his or her behavior and encouraged to express his or her point of view; punishment is used as a last resort;
- social role models: the child learns to do a variety of things properly; adults play a role of his or her moral models and pass on religious beliefs;
- encouragement to autonomy: adults, particularly parents, encourage the child to become independent, to search for help in difficult situations; they praise the child for autonomy and initiative;
- access to healthcare, education, welfare and public safety institutions: these services address those needs of the child that parents are not able to address;

Factors contained in category **I am** include the child's personal traits described as follows:

- loveable, attracting other people's attention: the child is aware that other people like and love him or her; the child wants to deserve this love by taking actions that are worth attention; the child maintains a proper balance between animation and calmness;
- loving, empathic, altruistic: the child loves other people and shows it in many ways, empathizes with and relieves other people's suffering and pain;
- proud of oneself: the child has a sense of importance and self-acknowledgement because he or she knows his or her strong and weak points; the child does not let other people belittle him or her; the child's self-trust and self-esteem let him or her manage successfully in difficult situations;

- independent and responsible: the child is capable of taking different actions and their consequences; the child has a sense of agency and accepts responsibility, acknowledges other people's control and responsibility;
- full of hope, faith and trust: the child believes that other people trust him or her but also that he or she trusts them; the child has a sense of good and evil, wants to multiply good, turns towards higher values;

Factors belonging to category **I can** include the child's social and interpersonal skills, aptly expressed by the following verbs:

- communicate: the child is able to communicate his or her thoughts and emotions towards others; the child can accurately interpret and understand other people's emotions, and responds to them;
- solve problems: the child can determine the core of the problem and plan its solution, negotiate solution options; the child can find creative solutions, with a certain measure of self-irony;
- cope with his or her own feelings and impulsiveness: the child is able to recognize and name his or her emotions and feelings, refrain from impulsive behaviors and those causing other people's pain;
- assess his or her own and other people's temperament: the awareness of his or her own traits and responses helps the child to behave adequately in many situations;
- establish interpersonal relationships based on trust: when in danger, the child is able to find somebody whom he or she would ask for help with solving internal or external conflicts.

A resilient child does not have to manifest all of the above-mentioned qualities, yet surely their broader range and higher level of intensity would guarantee a higher-quality psychological resilience. As Grotberg's studies show, only 38% of parents consciously foster resilience in their children; other children become resilient at high psychosocial costs.

Resilience of children with chronic conditions from the standpoint of positive psychology

Positive psychology is a relatively new current, both in the theory and practice of psychology – it was initiated in 1998 by M. Seligman, M. Csikszetmihalyi and R. Fowler. The founders of this sub-discipline modified the focus of psychology – its excessive concentration on deficits – to take a closer look also at assets in the functioning of man, in other words, they proposed a shift in the focus of psychological studies from the weakest points in the life of man to what makes it worth living. The overriding aim of positive psychology as a branch of knowledge and practice is then striving after a better and better understanding of not only abnormalities that may occur in human behavior, and man's negative responses to trauma but also, and perhaps more than anything else, of the process of man's adaptation to different life situations, of positive emotions, adaptive coping ways and hope (Gable, Haidt, 2005; Linley, Joseph, Harrington, Wood, 2006).

The ideas of positive psychology have quickly spread to the health psychology, rehabilitation psychology and clinical psychology, reinforcing their theoretical basis and outlining the new directions of studies. It turned out that the achievements of the new trend are intensely related to the theoretical and empirical findings of the above-mentioned sciences with regard to children. These relations have become clearly visible in the study of resilience – with post-traumatic growth and health-related quality of life of children and youth most often recognized as its indicators – and in the study of factors securing the development and functioning of children and youth in the case of external (e.g. poverty, violence, cataclysm) and internal (e.g. disability, severe somatic disease) dangers.

Post-traumatic growth refers to positive changes in the functioning of man resulting from experiencing traumatic events. Such changes usually include: discerning new opportunities in life, higher appreciation for life, improved social relations, an increased sense of one's personal power, and spiritual development. In the terminology used to describe those changes there are such expressions as: discovering meaning, flourishing, drawing strength from adversity or transformative coping (quoted after: Ogińska-Bulik, Juczyński, 2008). A study of post-traumatic growth in children and youth is rarely undertaken, most often because of methodological problems. L.P. Barakat, M.A. Alderfer and A.E. Kazak (2006) discovered that as many as 85% of teenagers suffering from cancer pointed out at least one positive change in themselves resulting from experiencing a difficult situation, and one-third of them could see four or more such changes. S. Phipps (2007), on the other hand, stresses a positive correlation of post-traumatic growth with optimism and self-evaluation, and its negative correlation with fear in tested groups of children with an oncological disease. According to M. Stępa (2006), one-third of youth suffering from asthma, diabetes or moderate and severe physical disability perceive a sense of their life situation in positive terms. Physically disabled youth is a group most often positively perceiving their health problem (48.33%), then there are youngsters suffering from asthma (35%), and finally diabetes (23.33%). Limitations and requirements resulting from health problems constitute a challenge for subjects; for some it is a chance to carry out new tasks, goals and values, for others – a specific kind of experience. The meaning ascribed to one's own disease, more than the knowledge of it or the concomitant emotions, determines the examined youth's adaptive difficulties. A negative meaning occurs together with externalizing difficulties, and particularly with a tendency towards problematic behaviors with predominant aggression. Youth discovering a meaning in their struggle with limitations and requirements that their disease entails, much more seldom manifest abnormalities in their social functioning. In recent years new studies have appeared (Zebrack, Chesler, 2002), showing a positive effect of a situation of cancer disease on the psychosocial development of youth. Young people undertake a reconstruction of their life goals, reinforce their resilience, build a positive attitude towards life, the attitude dominated by the acceptance of what life brings and tolerance towards other people. L.P. Barakat, E.R. Pulgaron, L.C. Daniel (2009), on the other hand, refer to various researchers whose findings show that children in cancer remission evaluate their life quality higher than their healthy peers, while children suffering from asthma, diabetes and cystic fibrosis ascribe a lower quality to their life.

According to L.P. Barakat, E.R. Pulgaron and L.C. Daniel (2009), among the factors protecting and reinforcing resilience in children and youth with chronic conditions are: self-esteem, hope and optimism, active coping, repressive adaptive style, family functioning and social support.

Self-esteem, in the opinion of A. Jakubik (1997), is a belief in an autonomous value of oneself and an expectation of its confirmation by other people and oneself. According to H. Grzegołowska-Klarkowska (1989), self-esteem constitutes a global feeling, a subjectively experienced global assessment of oneself. The development of self-esteem is related to two factors: self-evaluation in the areas important to the individual and an assessment of perceived relations with significant persons (Harter, 2005). The global self-esteem of children and youth with chronic illnesses does not differ significantly from that of their healthy peers. Lowering or inflating tendencies with regard to self-evaluation occur when young people face failures and negative emotions from other people (rejection and stigmatization). Moderately raised self-esteem enhances the realization of life goals and acquisition of social competences; it protects the person from fear, depression and asocial behaviors (e.g. avoiding, opposing, rebelling, egocentric behaviors). Positive self-esteem is recognized as the most important factor in the optimal functioning of the individual (Harter, 2005; Barakat, Pulgaron, Daniel, 2009).

Having hope is a fundamental condition of being a human. The losing or shattering of hope leads to the destruction of life. According to E. Fromm (2000), hope represents man's internal state that determines readiness for an intensive, though still unfulfilled, activity that would enable the person to achieve the fullness of life. It is such an internal state that makes the person follow "the inner voice," namely act, change oneself and the world always "for the better." Our life and the life of other people changes all the time, it is never the same, thus we also do change, we can overcome our weaknesses and limitations or give in to them. At every second of our life we can be stronger or weaker, wiser or dumber, bolder or more cowardly. Losing hope gives way to the indifference of the heart, hatred towards the world, desire to destroy it. V.E. Frankl (2009) by contrast believes that hope is a manifestation of the internal attitude of the individual and his or her will positively oriented towards life in general. It motivates man to accept what life brings, makes it possible to fight off the feeling of resignation or escape from life. Hope facilitates changes in the way we perceive our life situation, helps us to acquire the ability to interpret the world optimistically and to constantly improve the quality of our life. It is worth here to supplement Frankl's thoughts with M. Seligman's deliberations on optimism (1993). According to him, optimism helps man in four ways: it prevents a sense of helplessness and impotence, enhances our activeness when we have problems, and our aspiration to overcome them; it facilitates deep emotional relations with other people, protects us from too many adversities. The sources of optimism lie in the person's resourcefulness, positive attitude to life and the world, as well as in a style of explanation. The studies of hope and optimism in children and youth suffering from diseases that may lead to death or disability have shown that a higher level of hope and optimism is a predicator of effective adaptation to the limitations and discipline that the treatment and rehabilitation entail, of coping with pain and of higher expectations with regard to the process of education (Barakat, Pulgaron, Daniel, 2009).

Active coping includes effective ways of problem solving and a skillful search for and use of social support. The results of using such strategies depend on how they fit to the character of the problem, on the cognitive abilities and personality traits of children and youth, as well as on the duration of coping – avoidance strategies are most effective at short intervals of time, while problem-centered strategies – at longer ones. Emotional support plays an important role in active coping. Active coping enhances social adaptation, lowers the level of fear, reinforces self-esteem, relieves pain (Barakat, Pulgaron, Daniel, 2009; Pilecka, Fryt, 2011).

The essence of a repressive adaptive style lies in a low level of fear and a strong tendency to use defensive reactions and behaviors (avoidance, denial, withdrawal). This type of adaptation occurs in situations in which hardly controllable and non-modifiable stressors operate – e.g. in danger of disability or death. S. Phipps with a group of researchers (2006) pointed out that children suffering from cancer manifested a higher level of repressive adaptive style than healthy children. This dimension of functioning of children and youth with health and developmental problems has been poorly examined in empirical studies.

Family functioning is one of the most crucial determinants of the psychosocial development of every child. The subject literature highlights the importance of two dimensions: cohesion and adaptability, whose levels reveal the character of relations in the family and of the family with more distant circles of community. Cohesion refers to the emotional closeness of family members and at the same time their sense of autonomy within the family as a system. The relationship between this dimension of functioning and resilience of children is most often explored in the studies of active and affective family involvement and the specificity of interactions between parents and children. Adaptability of the family refers to its ability to modify its goals, principles, roles and leadership in order to maintain or reconstruct the inner balance in confrontation with serious dangers. Fostering resilience in children is particularly determined by two components of family adaptability: parental conduct also called a parenting style, and the modes of problem solving in view of the system of beliefs and values. Affective involvement refers to the degree to which family members value and manifest their interest in the actions of other family members. The intensity of this interest and the ways in which it is manifested are stressed. The development of resilience and healthy adaptation of children are related to the empathic involvement of other family members. An active involvement of family members in children's actions makes it possible to shape children's positive attitudes towards school, prevent their absence from school, help them achieve high marks and eliminate problematic behaviors. A shared system of values, beliefs and expectations, in the subject literature called a family schema, family world view or family cohesion, constitutes a significant indicator of family adaptability (quoted after: Sheridan, Eagle, Dowd, 2006). The family with a strong family schema looks at life realistically and does not expect prefect solutions for difficult situations. In its actions, such a family is more WE- than I-oriented. The members of a resilient family judge critical moments in the life of the family similarly, solve financial problems together, and organize their time together. They provide a lot of support to each other. Strong family resilience is a source of its each member's individual resilience. The very family itself, however, does need a formal and informal support of the external community with fostering its resilience through reinforcing the competences, strength and skills of its members and the whole family as a system.

The scope of the term *social support* is extremely broad and it includes diverse forms of help: sympathy, raising hope and encouragement, practical help, providing information, etc. A range of help and a number of people providing support are perceived as objective indicators of social support. In comparative studies of a network of social support for families with chronically sick and healthy children, no quantitative nor qualitative differences were found with regard to the size of the network, yet the studies proved its positive impact on the psychosocial adaptation of the child and his or her family. The network cannot be too dense (many persons providing support through mutual communication and action), as in such a case the activeness of its members disturbs the functioning of the family as a system. The activeness intensifies the system's cohesion to such a degree that it becomes a factor that curbs the independence and autonomy of family members and hinders expressing negative emotions by family members, especially their discontent with and a kind of disapproval of some aspects of family life. People providing informal support (more distant relatives, old and new friends) usually trigger sources of formal support, i.e. institutions launched to provide this kind of support, e.g. health and/or rehabilitation centers, associations.

Formal support refers to help that parents can get from institutions and professionals. In general parents expect reliable and understandable information on the disease or developmental problems of their child, as well as practical tips for nursing, care, up-bringing and rehabilitation. Parents differ in terms of their ability to understand and assimilate the information they are given, to formulate questions, as well as with regard to the modes of expressing their concerns and worries. Professionals should not only see to it that they inform parents in the way adequate to the parents' level of education and ability to understand the information they are given, but they should also ask extra questions to estimate the parents' needs with regard to the treatment, rehabilitation, care and up-bringing of the child.

Informal support comes from the family, friends, neighbors, as well as from organizations, associations whose members provide help voluntarily. The essence of this form of support lies in strong emotional bonds characterized by mutuality and maturity. A special role in the structure of informal support at early stages of child development is played by parents-veterans acting as consultants who share their experiences with persons at the beginning of their struggle with a new life situation caused by health problems of their daughter or son. At later stages of child development, especially in adolescence, great importance is attributed to peers' support that can be obtained through the child's relations with both sick and healthy peers. The two forms of support play an important role in fostering competences of the chronically ill child; they complement each other. Persons receiving informal support more effectively search for formal support because they learn where they can get it and how to use it. And the other way around – formal support reinforces informal forms of providing help characterized by mutuality and a lack of hierarchical structure. The atmosphere of egalitarianism and mutual respect lowers the level of fear and depression states, reinforces self-esteem, enhances the development of autonomy and a sense of agency, promotes mutual trust and openness, encourages expressing feelings (Pilecka, 2002).

Becoming a mature and well-functioning person as a developmental success

One of the most significant terms in positive psychology is *well-being* achieved through a *life well-lived*, i.e. active life focused on carrying out tasks and overcoming difficulties resulting from life changes. E. Diener, R.E. Lucas and S. Oishi (2012) define well-being as a cognitive and emotional assessment of our life, including both emotional responses to events and cognitive judgments of satisfaction with life. The assessment refers to six aspects of well-being: self-acceptance, life purpose, personal growth, control over the environment, positive relations with others and autonomy (Ryff, Singer, 2003).

Self-acceptance constitutes the most important dimension of well-being; it is manifested in a positive attitude towards oneself, feeling proud of oneself, accompanied with an awareness of one's strengths and weaknesses, successes and failures.

Another important dimension of well-being is having a life purpose that is defined by specific tasks resulting from undertaken social roles related to age, sex and sociocultural factors, as well as by the chosen hierarchy of values.

An aspect strongly related to having a life purpose is personal growth whose essence lies in the maximal actualization of one's total developmental potentials and special talents enhancing optimal functioning. A unique personal development very often results from battling against adversities and one's psychophysical limitations.

Control over the environment refers to coping with the surrounding reality in such a way that addressing one's needs and accomplishing personal standards is possible. Not only does it consist in controlling what is going on in the closest and further environment but also in engaging in the creation and nurturing of basic microenvironments and their mutual relations in the course of life.

This aspect is explicitly linked with the person's positive social relations being a source of not only pleasure and joy but also deep feelings and social support.

The last mentioned dimension – autonomy – stands for: the ability to manage one's behavior, make choices with one's own and other people's needs in view, and shape social relations based on mutuality

Well-being is presented here as a complex and multidimensional construct and as such has not been a subject of study of pediatric psychology so far, for many years, however, almost all of its aspects, as separate from one another areas of the functioning of children with chronic conditions, have been less or more directly described on the basis of empirical studies. Generalizing the findings of these studies it should be stated that most of the children strive after self-acceptance (Pilecka, 2002). In a situation of proper control over the course of the disease, ill children's self-regulatory competences are even higher than in the case of their healthy peers (Fryt, 2011); pediatric cancer survivors reconstruct their life goals (Zebrack, Chesler, 2002), and sometimes even transcendence expressed through their creative activeness (Pilecka, 2011).

In psychological literature several descriptions of a mature and well-functioning persons can be found. According to C.G. Jung (quoted after: Płużek, 2002), the first researcher to present the thesis that a human develops throughout his or her whole life, the most important traits of full humanness are: bestowing one's love upon oneself and others, realizing one's dignity and worth as well as the dignity of any other person, accepting responsibility for oneself and for others, and taking responsibility for good and evil in oneself and in other people. G. Allport (quoted after: Płużek, 2002), on the other hand, describes a mature person as characterized by such behaviors and attributes as: expanding one's personality, friendly contact with other people, emotional maturity, realistic attitude to life, talents and self-objectivization: insight and sense of humor, unifying life philosophy. A. Maslow (2006) ascribes many more traits to a mature person, i.e.: realistic perception of reality (a unique ability to discern what is fake, pretended and dishonest in all areas of life), self-acceptance, spontaneity, problem-centering, enduring loneliness with no self-cost and distress, autonomy, freshness of appreciation, peak experiences, sense of community with other people, modesty and respect, strong interpersonal relations, ethics (high moral standards), ability to distinguish between means and goals, sense of humor, creativity, resistance to cultural influences, imperfection, system of values, resolution of dichotomies (desires are in an accord with reason).

The diagram below illustrates the gist of the presented discussion:

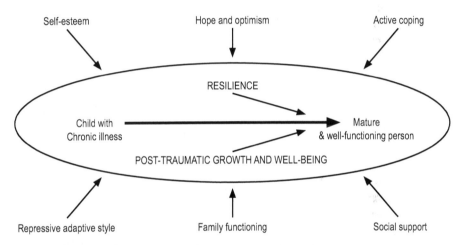

Figure 1. Developmental goal. Becoming a mature and well-functioning person

M. Stachel (2011), when analyzing a life situation of young women with physical disabilities, points out the following criteria that the women have to meet in order to achieve a full personal development: perceiving difficulties and limitations as challenges and tasks, accepting oneself the way one is, opening oneself to the world, a sense of being the subject of one's own life, having a life purpose or several life purposes, expanding the range of values. As the author writes, the process of personal growth requires an enormous effort and will to fight from persons afflicted with disability. Such a person has to come to terms with losing his or her physical fitness, accept oneself as a whole together with all the imperfections and deficits, open oneself to the world, introduce many changes into one's system of values, define one's life purposes and strive after their realization, but above all take control over one's own life that should be ran by disabled persons themselves, even though a presence and help of other persons is often necessary. It is worth noticing here that the system of values of the person with a somatic disease should also define this person's attitude towards suffering. If the attitude is positive and the person accepts suffering and learns to endure it, some day he or she will find meaning in it that will enhance the person's further work on oneself and his or her personal growth.

Having compared the conceptualization of psychological well-being with a description of a mature and well-functioning person, it can be stated that a human becomes such a person by achieving a full well-being at successive moments and situations of his or her life. In other words, psychological well-being determines the aspiration to become a mature and well- or optimally-functioning person.

The constant process of becoming a mature and well-functioning person – i.e. the person who perceives his or her limitations as tasks or challenges, who stays in communal closeness with others, who accepts oneself and who is aware of one's strengths and weaknesses, who is open to new experiences and to the world, who is the subject of his or her own life, who has got and carries out his or her life goals and expanded system of values – constitutes a fundamental goal of the psychosocial development of children and youth battling against the demands and limitations imposed on them by a chronic somatic disease. In the subject perspective, this process proceeds from an inevitable dependence on others towards a more and more dynamic self-creation. Psychological resilience (e.g. as formulated by E. Grotberg), post-traumatic growth and psychological well-being are regarded as direct determinants of this growth, or in other words – its psychological mechanisms. These determinants, on the other hand, are determined by protective factors of internal (self-esteem, hope and optimism, active coping and repressive adaptive style) and external character (family functioning and social support). It has to be added, though, that this process is possible only if the closest micro-environments of chronically ill children and youth (family, health and educational institutions) promote it through carrying out supportive actions, both informal (creating an emotional and motivating climate) and formal ones (psychoeducational, prophylactic and psychotherapeutic programs), in the context of favorable political solutions for healthcare and education.

References

Barakat, L.P., Pulgaron, E.R., Daniel, L.C. (2009). Positive Psychology in Pediatric Psychology. [In:] M.C. Roberts, R.G. Steele (Eds.). *Handbook of Pediatric Psychology*. New York–London: The Guilford Press.

Barakat, L.P., Alderfer, M.A., Kazak, A.E. (2006). Posttraumatic Growth in Adolescents Survivors of Cancer and Their Mothers and Fathers. *Journal of Pediatric Psychology*, 31, 413–419.

155

Diener, E., Lucas, R.E., Oishi, S. (2012). *Dobrostan psychiczny. Nauka o szczęściu i zadowoleniu z życia*. [W:] J. Czapiński (red.). *Psychologia pozytywna*. Warszawa: Wydawnictwo Naukowe PWN.

Frankl, V.E. (2009). *Człowiek w poszukiwaniu sensu*. Warszawa: Wydawnictwo „Czarna Owca".

Fromm, E. (2000). *Rewolucja nadziei*. Poznań: Dom Wydawniczy REBIS.

Fryt, J. (2011). S*amoregulacja i funkcjonowanie poznawcze u dzieci z astmą i cukrzycą typu 1 w okresie późnego dzieciństwa*. Niepublikowana praca doktorska pod kierunkiem W. Pileckiej. Kraków: Instytut Psychologii UJ.

Gable, S.L., Haidt, J. (2005). What (and Why) is Positive Psychology? *Review of General Psychology*, 9, 103–110.

Grotberg, E. (2000). *Zwiększenie odporności psychicznej – wzmacnianie sił duchowych*. Warszawa: Wydawnictwo Akademickie „Żak".

Grzegołowska-Klarkowska, H. (1989). *Determinanty mechanizmów obronnych osobowości: studium empiryczne z perspektywy psychologii poznawczej*. Wrocław: Wydawnictwo Naukowe PAN.

Handbook of resilience in children (2006). New York: Springer.

Harter, S. (2005). *The Development of Self-Representations during Childhood and Adolescence*. [In:] Leary, M.R., Tangney, J.P. (Eds.). *Handbook of self and identity*. New York: The Guilford Press.

Jakubik, A. (1997). *Zaburzenia osobowości*. Warszawa: Wydawnictwo Naukowe PZWL.

Jordan, J.V. (2006). *Relational Resilience in Girls*. [In:] S. Goldstein, R.B. Brooks (Eds.).

Linley, P.A., Joseph, S., Harrington, S., Wood, A.M. (2006). Positive Psychology: Past, Present and (possible) Future. *Journal of Positive Psychology*, 1, 3–16.

Maslow, A. (2006). *Motywacja i osobowość*. Warszawa: Wydawnictwo Naukowe PWN.

Newacheck, P.W., Taylor, W.R. (1992). Childchood Chronic Illness: Prevalence, Severity, and Impact. *American Journal of Public Health*, 82 (3), 364–371.

Noll, R.B., Kupst, M.J. (2007). The Psychological Impact of Pediatric Cancer Hardiness: The Exception or the Rule?*Journal of Pediatric Psychology*, 32, 1089–1098.

O'Dougherty-Wright, M., Masten, A.S. (2006). *Resilience Processes in Development*. [In:] S. Goldstein, R.B. Brooks (Eds.). *Handbook of resilience in children*. New York: Springer.

Ogińska-Bulik, N., Juczyński, Z. (2008). *Osobowość, stres a zdrowie*. Warszawa: Difin.

Phipps, S. (2007). Adaptive Style in Children with Cancer: Implications for a Positive Psychology Approach. *Journal of Pediatric Psychology*, 32, 1055–1066.

Phipps, S., Larson, S., Long, A., Rai, S.N. (2006). Adaptive Style and Symptoms of Posttraumatic Stress in Children with Cancer and their Parents. *Journal of Pediatric Psychology*, 31, 298–309.

Pilecka, W. (2002). *Przewlekła choroba somatyczna w życiu i rozwoju dziecka*. Kraków: Wydawnictwo Uniwersytetu Jagiellońskiego.

Pilecka, W. (2011). *Zmaganie się dziecka z przewlekłą chorobą somatyczną – od radzenia sobie do transcendencji*. [W:] B. Antoszewska (red.). *Dziecko przewlekle chore – problemy medyczne, psychologiczne i pedagogiczne*. Toruń: Wydawnictwo Edukacyjne „AKAPIT".

Pilecka, W., Fryt, J. (2011). *Teoria stresu dziecięcego*. [W:] W. Pilecka (red.). *Psychologia zdrowia dzieci i młodzieży. Perspektywa kliniczna*. Kraków: Wydawnictwo Uniwersytetu Jagiellońskiego.

156

Płużek, Z. (2002). *Psychologia pastoralna*. Kraków: Wydawnictwo Instytut Teologiczny Księży Misjonarzy.

Ryff, C.D., Singer, B. (2003). *The Role Emotions on Pathways to Positive Health*. [In:] R.J. Davidson, K.R. Scherer, H.H. Goldschmit (Eds.). *Handbook of Affective Sciences*. New York: Oxford University Press.

Seligman, M.P. (1993). *Optymizmu można się nauczyć*. Poznań: Wydawnictwo Media Rodzina.

Seligman, M.P., Csikszentmihalyi, M. (2000). Positive Psychology: An Introduction. *American Psychologist*, 56, 216–217.

Sheridan, S.M., Eagle, J.W., Dowd, S.E. (2006). Families as Contexts for Children's Adaptation. [In:] S. Goldstein, R.B. Brooks (Eds.). *Handbook of Resilience in Children*. New York: Springer.

Stachel, M. (2011). *Niepełnosprawność ruchowa jako sytuacja graniczna w osobowym rozwoju kobiety*. Niepublikowana praca doktorska pod kierunkiem W. Pileckiej. Kraków: Instytut Psychologii UJ.

Stępa, M. (2006). *Postawa wobec własnej choroby przewlekłej a przystosowanie społeczne młodzieży*. Niepublikowana praca doktorska pod kierunkiem W. Pileckiej. Kraków: Instytut Pedagogiki UJ.

Thompson, R.J. Jr., Gustafson, K.E. (1996). *Adaptation to Chronic Childhood Illness*. Washington: APA.

Tyszkowa, M. (1986). *Zachowanie się dzieci szkolnych w sytuacjach trudnych*. Warszawa: Wydawnictwo Naukowe PWN.

Wyman, P.A., Sandler, I., Wolchik, S., Nelson, K. (2000). *Resilience as Cumulative Competence Promotion and Stress Protection: Theory and Intervention*. [In:] D. Cicchetti, J. Rappaport, I. Sandler, R.P. Weissberg (Eds.). *The Promotion of Wellness in Children and Adolescents*. Washington: DC: Child Welfare League of America.

Zebrack, B.J., Chesler, M.A. (2002). Quality of Life in Childhood Cancer Survivors. *Psycho-Oncology*, 11, 132–141.

Wojciech Otrębski, Barbara Czuba
The John Paul II Catholic University of Lublin
Institute of Psychology

COPING WITH STRESS AMONGST FAMILIES WITH CHILDREN SUFFERING FROM CHRONIC PSYCHOSOMATIC DISEASES – RECOMMENDATIONS FOR PSYCHOPROPHYLACTIC ACTIONS

Abstract

For over fifty years, psychosomatic medicine has been an organized branch of science. The crucial role in psychosomatic disorders is played by emotional factors which elongate the changes in the functioning of the immune and endocrynological systems (Szewczyk, 2001). Prolonged preservation of certain emotions leads to illnesses. Among skin conditions, atopic dermatitis proves to be a growing problem. It is chronically, troublesome and difficult to cure completely and its causes and occurrences is linked with mental conditions (Januszewska, 2001; Nowicki, 2009).

Literary analysis show that the disease occurring within the family system is one of the most acutely working stress stimuli for this family (Hoes, 1997; Plopa, 2004). Research conducted on patients with skin dermatitis (Benea, Muresian, Manolache, Robu, Diaconu, 2001) show health deterioration usually linked with accumulation of stressful events. These patients signalled a feeling of loneliness in the family and being severely punished by their parents. Polish research in this field were mainly conducted on adolescent patients suffering from acne and atopic dermatitis, and who came from families where the bond between the child and parent was too strong and the child's need to subordinate and meet the parent's demand, caused the symptoms of the illness to become more acute. (Tuszynska-Bogucka, 2007).

From the point of view of psychoprophylactics and because of the aforementioned facts, it seems necessary to analyze ways of dealing with stress and correct functioning of the family system where there is a child suffering from psychosomatic diseases.

Key words: coping, psychosomatic disease, childhood, prophylactics

Introduction

According to salutogenesis, health and illness create a continuum in which every person holds a certain (Pilecka, 2011). Health and development of children and adolescents are conditioned by the quality of the surrounding environment. Research results of the Fogarty Foundation (Pilecka, 2011, p. 8), show that 10 to 18% of children and adolescents up to 21 years of age, show full and untouched psychophysical fitness (za: Pilecka, 2011), hence attention to health and development of children should be the most important predicator to their high standard living as adults.

Issues concerning children's and adolescents' health, are proving to become of utmost interest through the world, as is understanding the problems connected with the primary and natural living environment, which is family, and its influence on a single. A family that takes care of an ill person and helps him get back to health, is often forced to change their plans.

Thus, a family often makes internal changes to help the ill person to regain full fitness. It can be said that on some level, the family is ill along with the child and that the situation of the patient cannot be looked upon without paying attention to the family situation (Swietochowski, 2008). Because of that, illness within a family should not be disregarded and lack of sufficient data motivates to deepen the specialist knowledge in this field.

While regarding the issues concerning characteristics of psychosomatic diseases, a certain inquests of developmental problems can be observed, namely that unexpected occurrence of an illness is not accepted by members of the family. It puts the family in a situation where it has to activate special abilities to reorganize its structure and function to meet the demands of the illness. In case of a persons' sickness, the family is the primary environment of that person and the entire family system has to struggle with it, creating special conditions for the patient and ensuring socio-emotional support.

A theoretical basis for these dissertations is on one hand the theory of systems and on the other stress theory, as an experience which is the consequence of the met difficulties and also up to date knowledge of the clinical picture of psychosomatic diseases which are allergies. Research conducted within these families make it possible to understand and describe the problems and difficulties faced by parents of chronically psychosomatically sick children. The aim of this thesis is to enrich the current state of awareness which may prove helpful in organizing suitable therapeutic influence.

Specification of chronic psychosomatic diseases on the example of allergies – literary analysis

It is estimated that even every third person on the planet suffers from allergies. These are usually children and young people. 10–25% of the population, which is even 500 millions people, suffers from hay fever. Depending on the country, 1–18% of the population develops asthma. 300 millions people in the world suffer from it. Atopic dermatitis is a typical condition for the early age of life as in 15–20% of cases it concerns children and only 1–3% adults. (*Nature Reviews Immunology*, 2006).

The results of ECAP program have provided valid data concerning the frequency of allergies in Poland (Samel-Kowalik et al., 2009). 22 700 people from 9 regions of the country took part in the program. Depending on the age, hay fever was present in 22–25% of the cases, asthma in 9–11% and atopic dermatitis in 4–9% (*Epidemiologia chorób alergicznych w Polsce*, 2009).

As the research results indicate, there is still much to do in Poland. The basis for taking action should be further, deepened analysis and research concerning how parents cope with their child's psychosomatic disease. This will help build a rational program addressed to the sick and their families, places of work and a widely recognized variety of medical environments.

An illness can disorganize the former functioning of the family system but is "being experienced by every member of that family as it demands placing oneself in a different role, undertake different actions which would be the most suitable as a reaction to the experienced stress" (Buczynski, 1999, p. 52).

For a psychosomatically sick person, the time of duration and intensity of the illness is important. In case of infectious diseases, limitations of everyday functioning are usually not severe and regaining health nearly full.

The most severe and long lasting obstacles in everyday functioning are linked with chronic diseases, which are usually untreatable and often lead to permanent loss of health. Additionally, they limit or make it impossible to be self-efficient. Characteristics of a chronic disease are longer duration, less acute course and irreversibility of the changes (Pilecka, 2002). A chronic disease may influence a family in two ways. On the one hand it may prove to be a factor which puts the family's integrity in danger and on the other hand the demand for rehabilitation may reintegrate it (Radochoński, 1987; Obuchowska, 1991; Kawczyńska-Butrym, 2001). According to Pilecka (2001), the dependency between the development of an ill child, the illness' course and the influence of the family system create a chain of mutual interaction with constant feedback. The researcher suggests that good family atmosphere favours effective rehabilitation of the patient. Also because a psychosomatic diseases, the entire scheme of relations within the family may change as well as the financial situation which is due to long-lasting costs of medication intake.

There have always been discussions concerning the definition of psycho-somatic diseases. A psychosomatic disease proves a challenge for modern day medicine as to what to treat: the symptoms of the disease or its psychological background? (Luban-Plozza, 1995; Budzyna-Dawidowski et al., 2000; Szew-czyk, 2006). Currently, it is possible to distinguish two main stands in this case. On the one hand it is the biomedical approach in which the physical condition of a person influences and is modified by his psychical state. On the other hand it is the general theory of systems which constitutes a starting point for system family therapies.

It is an interesting fact that the system approach tries to understand the psy-chosomatic disease in the context of family relations. A psychosomatic symptom has its meaning and after its decoding it transpires that it comprises of a bio-logical and emotional component. In this approach, a psychosomatic disorder is a warning sign which must be understood as a disorder which influences the per-son suffering from it as well as his environment. (Luban-Plozza, 1995; Pilecka, 2002; Szewczyk, 2006).

As the therapeutic works of the author of the psychosomatic system family concerning children suffering from diabetes – Minuchina (1975), regardless of good medical care, some children experienced complications. It transpired that these children came from families characterized by entanglement, overprotec-tiveness, strict rules and a weak ability to resolve or to avoid conflicts. They were also characterized by triangulation which means engaging a third party into the conflict, which in turn poses a threat to a two person relation.

According to Minuchin (1975), the disease and the family's attitude towards it, organizes his family in a way that influences how the child reacts to the ill-ness. The actions of the family trigger physiological factors, which in turn influ-ence deterioration of the disease.

Other researchers, such as Horney (1926: after Namysłowska, 2003, p. 36), put emphasis on cultural factors in the development of psychosomatic disorders. According to them, the theory of systems is the most useful one when it comes to understanding the creating of the course of psychosomatic disorders. According to this theory, pathological behaviours are examined in categories of the entire system and the sickness of one family member indicates a problem for the whole family system (Namysłowska, 2003). The cause of many stress related occur-rences may be the result of bad treatment of one another within the family, which in turn may cause or worsen psychosomatic symptoms (Pilecka, 2002). These symptoms may cause unfavourable changes in family interactions and even gen-erate adverse events in terms of burdening. Reactions of a family system to-wards a chronic disease of its member, do not give a straightforward answer to the question of its true influence on the family.

However, reactions of the family which are aimed at mainly the state of bal-ance, are becoming visible. In fear of altering the scheme of every day function-ing, the family may strengthen the feeling of uncertainty and lead to additional burdening, limit communication, trigger conflicts or suppress (Januszewska, 2001; Pilecka, 2002; Namysłowska, 2003; Tuszyńska-Bogucka, 2007).

Research prove that mothers more than fathers are burdened with caring for a sick child and this is mainly linked with bigger distress concerned with the illness rather than that concerning the rehabilitation process (Wyczesany, 2000). Research on expressing emotions within 32 families with children between the ages of 5 and 12 suffering from asthma, was carried out Hermanns, Florin, Dietrich and associates (1989: after Garthland, Day et al., 1999, p. 275). The findings show bigger criticism among fathers which was in turn linked to the children's absence from school. A negative correlation between the time devoted to children by fathers and the occurrence of illness symptoms, has been noticed. Different conclusions were reached by Schobinger and Florin (Ostrowski, 1995, p. 99) while examining 28 families of children with asthma. The authors deduced that both mothers and fathers of asthmatic children, more often show a critical attitude towards their children than parents of healthy ones and this criticism is linked with a more acute course asthma. However, the mothers proved to be more critical. Furthermore, the fathers' bigger engagement to rehabilitation and spending time with the sick child causes the course of the symptoms to be more benign. One can assume that because of the mothers' bigger burdening with their children's' health problems and their states of exhaustion, they become critical and anxious more often. Above that, a child with an allergy may more frequently than a healthy one, be hyperactive and show behaviour disorders.

Inter-family interactions have also become subject of interest for Norwegian long-term researches, carried out between 1987 and 1997 on a group of 100 children suffering from atopic dermitis (Gustafsson, 1997). In light of their outcome, it has been stated that dysfunctional interactions occurred within 37% of the examined families. These were families of newborns with early signs of whizzing cough. This dysfunctional problem was linked with how advanced the illness of the asthmatic children was when the improper interactions were indeed stated.

This group was also characterized by over protectiveness. Furthermore, the results show that fear caused by children having symptoms of whizzing cough, have a negative influence on family relations. Dysfunctional behaviour patterns cause the occurrence of tension within the family and they reduce the abilities to cope with problems and thus become risk factors of the disease to continue and occurrence of acute form of asthma.

A child's emotional development is constituted not by the specification of the illness itself but by the behaviour of people from their immediate surroundings. If, because of them, the situation of the illness is interpreted as danger and triggers an emotional type of coping, then the malfunctions in the child's existence will intensify. If parents can treat the demands and shortcomings connected with the child's illness in the category of challenges or tasks, then their behaviours will enable the child to keep internal balance and develop mechanisms of emotional control both in parents and children. (Pilecka, 2011).

Scientific research and all therapeutic doings should concern the child in the context of its relations with their closest environments (Pilecka, 2011). It has been observed that patients suffering from skin conditions show a larger number of stressful life situations that took place in the time preceding the illness. The results of the researches conducted on patients with atopic derimitis (Benea, Muresian, Manolache, Robu, Diaconu, 2001), indicate deterioration usually linked with an accumulation of stressful occurrences, especially concerning interpersonal relations. Literary analysis proves that sudden traumatic events like trauma may cause spot baldness. It has been indicated that in the period preceding the occurrence of symptoms, many of the sick went through psychical trauma or a difficult time incident. (Gupta, Gupta, Watteel, 1996).

The role of economic and social status, the size of the family, the way of feeding infants or pollution play significant roles in some researches, whereas in others they are not of much importance (Romanska et al., 2006). Romanska, along with her co-researchers, agrees that exposure to bacterial, animal and plant allergens in early childhood, has a positive impact on atopic disease prophylactic.

In accordance with the hygienic hypothesis, an atopic outburst occurs more often among children who have no siblings and are less often in danger of common inflammation. This hypothesis is not backed up by researches conducted by other authors, for example German ones, like: Zutavern, Hirsch, Leupold, (after: Romanska et al., 2006, p. 230).

They have not indicated a positive correlation between atopic dermitis and the size of the family. Contrary conclusions were introduced by Hungarian: Sebok, Schneider, Parangi (after: Romanska et al., 2006, p. 230), according to whom, an atopic outburst statistically concerned single children more often. However, the Hungarian researches did not take into account the fact of the child attending kindergarten and the frequency of common inflammations occurring.

A significant majority of theoretical and empiric analyses show the influence of a chronically sick person on the functioning of the entire family, although in subject literature the influence of a child's disease on marriage and its stability was seldom undertook. Giving birth to a chronically sick or a handicapped child may prove to be a factor both cementing and disintegrating a marriage. (Januszewska, 2001; Pilecka, 2002; Namysłowska, 2003; Tuszyńska-Bogucka, 2007).

In assessing the quality of life of families with children who suffer from atopic dermitis, the DFIQ (*Dermatitis Family Impact Questionnaire*) questionnaire was used. It assesses the influence of the child's illness on 10 spheres of family life, including: additional duties, preparing special meals, sleeping disorders amongst members of family caused by the sick child's symptoms. The questionnaire also takes into account the way of spending free time, additional expenses due to the sickness, the feeling of exhaustion amongst parents and the emotional relations amongst other members of the family (Teresiak et al., 2006). Lowering the standard of life concerns also the families of those suffering from atopic dermitis. A sick child sets higher standards for its loved ones, it needs specialist

care consisting of preparing a special diet, skin care, help in bathing and dressing and so on.

Frequent visits to the doctor are the cause of parents being made redundant. Subduing to rules and limitations leads to exhaustion and sleeping disorders. The sickness may cause a family crisis in the form of altering emotional ties. It often comes to them being either loosened or deepened. They are however dependent on the acuteness of skin irritation. As research have show, improvement of clinical condition of the sick child influences the improvement of the quality of family life (Teresiak et al., 2006; Lewis-Jones, 2006).

Sometimes taking care of a person suffering from atopic deritis forces restriction or resignation from professional work (Teresiak et al., 2006). Lack of pleasing effects of treating the sick person may lead to two extremes concerning the sick, especially if it is a child. This can be excessive concentration and sacrifice or indifference and helplessness. Overprotective parents try to exclude the child's independence by solving all problems for the child. This leads to lowering the child's self-confidence and ability to cope with difficult situations. Concentrating mainly on the sick child may cause conflicts when it comes to relations with other siblings who start to feel jealous or have the feeling of being rejected. Submissiveness towards the sick child may cause egocentrism to root itself and lessen sensitivity towards the needs of other family members. (Teresiak et al., 2006; Lewis-Jones, 2006).

The parents' attitude and personality have a crucial role in the child's personal development. It has been indicated that the family situation correlates with the level of intensifying the course of the sickness and the itching sensation. Mutual relations between the sick child and the family is crucial in curing atopic dermitis (Januszewska, 2001).

In the forties and fifties of the 20th century it has been discovered that atopic dermitis occurred more frequently among children who were rejected by mothers (Tuszyńska-Bogucka, 2007) or treated by them in a hostile or strict way. Other researches (Palos, Ring, 1984) suggest that parents of the sick children often suffered from emotional tension, a feeling of guilt and presented behaviours typical of over protectiveness. Sometimes this correlation showed these children's complete helplessness and inability to make their own, even petty, decisions.

Ways of dealing with stress amongst families with children suffering from chronic psychosomatic diseases – an overview of researches

The notion of adjusting to the sickness is directly linked to the problem of functioning of a family and ways of coping with the sickness. However, one must state that there exists no single definition of 'coping' with a chronic disease. According to Radochonski (1987), an adaptive system of the family coping with the illness is being adopted, which in turn is a process of mutual influence of abilities and sources as well as seeing elements that comprise a stressful situation and also emotional and behavioural reactions occurring in the family which struggles to regain its functioning balance (Radochoński, 1987). Stress factors influencing the family are of different backgrounds and cause specific changes in everyday life. They force a new division in duties, a change in the way of spending free time and master new, previously unknown abilities.

Stress is a recognized factor that provokes and sharpens the symptoms of psoriasis (Pietrzyk, 2006; Tuszyńska-Bogucka, 2007; Krasowska, Tuszyńska-Bogucka 2006).

Sudden, shattering events or recurring small burdens, escalate the symptoms that come with this disease. It has also a significant impact on causing and sustaining or worsening diseases such as prurigo, itch, too much sweating and eczema (Juszkiewicz-Borowiec, 1999). The percentage of people who suffered a disease which was preceded by a traumatically event is estimated at 10% to 68% (Tuszynska-Bogucka, 2007).

In works examining emotional reactions of parents to their children being diagnosed with chronic psychosomatic disease, the findings show that the occurrence of strong negative emotions. However some researchers suggest that parents deal with the child's disease differently and describe their emotions differently (Kerr, 2004).

Initially after Lazarus (1986), two form sort his reaction were distinguished: those aimed at the problem and those aimed at their own emotions. Later, coping concentrated on avoiding a meaning a consisting of using social support, was taken into account. The main role in Lazarus' concept is played by recognition assessment and transaction as a certain way of a single person functioning in relation with his or her surroundings.

Recognition assessment of a subject concerning balance between abilities and demands decides if the transaction is a stressful one.

His assessment is also a source of emotional reactions when faced with stress and also determines a stressful situation. One of the accusations that can be aimed at Lazarus' and Folkmans' concept (1986) is taking into account the timing context.

Hence, new concepts of dealing with stress take into account the time of occurrence of a stressful event. An example of it can be a classification proposed by Schwarzer and Taubert (1999), who distinguish 4 types in its occurrence:

(1) reactive which aims at compensating the pain nor loss;

(2) anticipative aimed at the event which is to occur in the near future;

(3) preventive linked with gathering reserves allowing to lessen the outcomes of future stressful events;

(4) proactive which concerns doping as special in the context of health requires a wider explanation.

Proactive coping with stress comprises 'autonomic and independent setting of goals which are a challenge and their consequent realization' (Schwarzer, Taubert, 1999, p. 86). So understood coping is aimed at motivating people to set ambitious goals and aspiring to their realization.

The main triggering force of his concept is searching for a challenge which is eased by the feeling of self-efficiency.

While Lazarus and Folkman (1986) state that coping is a process, other authors see it in categories of general disposition which is a way or strategy of coping. Research results on ways of parents coping with stress caused by cancer, which were conducted by Barbarin, Huges, Mesler in the eighties of the 19th century, allowed the identification of eight styles of coping with a difficult situation, concentrated on solving practical problems concerned with the child's curing process, searching for help outside of the family, sustaining the emotional balance, leaning on religion, staying optimistic, contradicting the diagnosis and accepting the situation.

Coping with stress within a family touched upon with a chronic disease includes three types of strategies (Olson et al., 1985). The first group is based on concentrating on family life and giving meaning to the disease. Another is based on maintain social life and professional perfecting, which favours good mental and physical feeling amongst family members. The third concentrates on supporting contacts with the medical staff and information flow with the parents of other children suffering from a similar disease. According to Olson (1985), there exist five groups of strategies of dealing with a difficult situation. These are: seeking social support, changing the definition of a stressful situation to a one possible to accept, seeking spirituals support, making use of help of institutions and organizations. The researches of Ochojska and Radochonski (1997), indicate that utmost importance, when it comes to dealing with a situation caused by a disease, is given to institutional help.

Summary

The frequency of allergies occurring around the world is growing and currently from 30% to 40% of the population suffers from it. It mainly concerns young people so it is only expected that at a later age the problems concerning allergies will deepen. More and more frequently, it can be observed that the occurrence of complex allergies in which bring prone to more than one allergen occurs and the disease affects more organs. The outcome here is a bigger number of people falling ill which in turn enforces more funds being given to public health institutions in order to cope with it. It can be foreseen that allergies will occur more frequently along with growing pollution and higher temperatures. This in consequence may lead to an increase in the number of diseases, deterioration of the quality of life, complications and a higher death toll as well as economic costs on the part of the patient.

From materials and analyses gathered, it transpires that patterns of paternal behaviour causes the occurrence of tension within families and reduce the abilities of coping with problems and thus become the risk factors of the disease to elongate itself. Researches concerning this topic show that the complexity and sudden occurrence of a disease causes the family to have interpersonal, existential, intellectual and instrumental problems (Radochonski, 1997; Pietrzyk, 2006).

The analysis of researches concerning dealing with difficult situation which is a child's disease, shows that coping with stress is usually viewed as a style or strategy. However, a chronic disease is not something 'finished' and thus coping with stress seen as a process, enables a deeper analysis of this phenomenon. (after: Heszen-Niejodek, 2000; Pisula, 2007). Currently, there are no researches which full show the process of how parents with chronically, psychosomatically sick children, cope with stress. In the overview of literature, the need of a more integrated approach surfaces, concerning both diagnostic and therapeutic issues. It is necessary to raise the level of social awareness concerning allergies and their prevention. Furthermore, educating medical care staff, concerning not only allergy departments but more importantly enabling cooperation with specialists from different fields in order to integrate caring for the sick person. It may however be anticipated that in face of the growing number of people falling ill, these shortcomings will soon be remedied.

References

Benea, V., Muresian, D., Manolache, L., Robu, E., Diaconu, J.D. (2001). Stress and atopic dermatitis. *Dermatology and Psychosomatics*, 2(4), 205–207.

Buczyński, L.F. (1999). *Rodzina z dzieckiem chorym na białaczkę*, Lublin: Wydawnictwo Katolickiego Uniwersytetu Lubelskiego.

Budzyna-Dawidowski, P., Barbaro de, B., Furgał, M. (2000). Podejście systemowe w diagnozie i leczeniu chorób psychosomatycznych. Systemowe rozumienie chorób psychosomatycznych. *Psychoterapia*, 3 (114), 41–58.

Epidemiologia chorób alergicznych w Polsce (2009). http://www.ecap.pl (accessed 12.09.2012).

Garthland, H.J., Day, H.D. (1999). Family Predictors of the Incidence of Children's Asthma Symptoms: Expressed Emotions, Medications, Parent Contact and Life Events. *Journal of Clinical Psychology*, 1999, 55, 573–584.

Gupta, M.A., Gupta, A.K. (1997). Psychodermatology: An update. *Journal of the American Academy of Dermatology*, 34, 1030–1046.

Heszen-Niejodek, I. (2000). *Stres i radzenie sobie – główne kontrowersje*. [W:] I. Heszen-Niejodek, Z. Ratajczak, (red.). *Człowiek w sytuacji stresu* (12–44). Katowice: Wydawnictwo Uniwersytetu Śląskiego.

Hoes, M.J.A.J.M (1997). Adverse life events and psychosomatic disease. *Current Opinion in Psychiatry*, 10(6), 462–465.

Januszewska, E. (2001). *Psychosomatyczne aspekty choroby skóry (neurodermitis)*. [W:] L. Szewczyk, A. Kulik (red.). *Wybrane zagadnienia z psychologii klinicznej i osobowości. Psychosomatyka* (79–96). Lublin: Towarzystwo Naukowe Katolickiego Uniwersytetu Lubelskiego.

Juszkiewicz-Borowiec, M. (1999). Udział stresu w etiopatogenezie wybranych chorób skóry. *Przegląd Dermatologiczny*, 86(1), 61–65.

Kawczynska-Butrym, Z. (2001). *Rodzina – Zdrowie – Choroba. Koncepcje i praktyka pielęgniarstwa rodzinnego*. Lublin: CZELEJ Sp. z o.o.

Kerr, L.M., Harrison, M.B., Medves, J., Tranmer, J. (2004). Supportive care needs of parents of children with cancer: Transition From Diagnosis to Treatment. *Oncology Nursing Forum*, rd. 36, no. 6, 116–126.

Krasowska, D., Tuszynska-Bogucka, W. (2006). Ocena wybranych aspektów osobowości i poziomu oraz poziomu stresu i stylu radzenia sobie ze stresem lęku u chorych na liszaj płaski. *Przegląd Dermatologiczny*, 94(2), 265–272.

Lazarus, R.S. (1986). Paradygmat stresu i radzenia sobie. *Nowiny Psychologiczne*, 3, 4, 2–39.

Lewis-Jones, S. (2006). Quality of life and childhood atopic dermatitis: the misery of living with childhood eczema. *International Journal of Clinical Practice*. 60(8), 984–992.

Luban-Plozza, B., Poldinger, W., Kroger, F., Wasilewski, B. (1995). *Zaburzenia Psychosomatyczne w praktyce lekarskiej*. Warszawa: Wydawnictwo Lekarskie PZWL.

Minuchin, S., Baker, L., Rosman, B.L, Liebman, R., Milman, L., Tood, T.C. (1975). A conceptual model of psychosomatic illness in children: Family organization and family therapy. *Arch. Gen. Psychiatry*, 32, 1031–1038.

Namysłowska, I. (2003). *System rodzinny a zaburzenia psychosomatyczne*. [W:] L. Szewczyk, M. Skowronska (red.). *Zaburzenia psychosomatyczne u dzieci i młodzieży* (35–48), Warszawa: Wydawnictwo EMU.

Nature Reviews Immunology (2006). www.alergie.mp.pl

Nowicki, R. (2009). Co nowego w leczeniu atopowego zapalenia skóry? *Postępy Dermatologii i Alergologii*, 24(5), 350–353.

Obuchowska, I. (1991). *Dziecko niepełnosprawne w rodzinie*, Warszawa: Wydawnictwa Szkolne i Pedagogiczne.

Ochojska, D., Radochonski, M. (1997). Choroba w rodzinie: Style zmagania się z sytuacją trudną, „Problemy Rodziny", 5/6, 39–43.

Olson, D.H, Mc Cubbin, I.H., Barnes, H., Larsen, A., Muxen, M., Wilson, M. (1985): *Family inventories*, Minnessota: University of Minnesota.

Ostrowski, T.M. (1995). *Mechanizm zaprzeczania w procesie zmagania się z chorobą.* [W:] D. Kubacka-Jasiecka (red.). *Wybrane problemy zmagania się ze stresem*, (123–138), Kraków: Wydawnictwo Uniwersytetu Jagiellońskiego.

Palos, E., Ring, J. (1984). Psychosomatic aspects of parent – child relations in atopic egzema of childhood. *Archives of Dermatological Research*, 276, 256.

Pietrzyk, A. (2006). *Ta choroba w rodzinie*, Kraków: Oficyna Wydawnicza IMPULS.

Pilecka, W. (2002). *Przewlekła choroba somatyczna w życiu i rozwoju dziecka*. Kraków: Wydawnictwo Uniwersytetu Jagiellońskiego.

Pilecka, W. (2011). *Psychologia zdrowia dzieci i młodzieży*. Kraków: Wydawnictwo Uniwersytetu Jagiellońskiego.

Plopa, M. (2004). *Psychologia rodziny: teoria i badania*. Elbląg: Wydawnictwo EWSH.

Radochonski, M. (1987). *Choroba a rodzina*. Rzeszów: WSP.

Romanska-Gocka, K., Gocki, J., Placek, W., Zegarska, B. (2006). Rola bariery skórnej, wybranych czynników środowiskowych i karmienia piersią w atopowym zapaleniu skóry. *Postępy Dermatologii i Alergologii*, 23(5), 228–233.

Samel-Kowalik, P., Lipiec, A., Tomaszewska, A., Raciborski, F., Walkiewicz, A., Lusawa, A., Borowicz, J., Gutowska-Slesik, J., Samolinski, B. (2009). Występowanie alergii i astmy w Polsce – badanie ECAP. Gazeta Farmaceutyczna, 3, 32–34.

Schwarzer, R., Taubert, S. (1999) Radzenie sobie ze stresem: wymiary i procesy. *Promocja Zdrowia. Nauki Społeczne i Medycyna*, 17, 72–92.

Szewczyk, L. (2001). *Psychobiologiczne mechanizmy zaburzeń psychosomatycznych u dzieci i młodzieży*. [W:] L. Szewczyk, A. Kulik (red.): *Wybrane zagadnienia z psychologii klinicznej i osobowości. Psychosomatyka*. Lublin: Towarzystwo Naukowe Katolickiego Uniwersytetu Lubelskiego.

Szewczyk, L. (2006). Patomechanizm i symptomatologia zaburzeń psychosomatycznych. *Alma Mater*, 59(2), 104–109.

Świętochowski, W. (2008). *Zastosowanie systemowej terapii rodzinnej w leczeniu chorób somatycznych*. [W:] L. Szewczyk, A. Kuklik (red.). *Problemy psychosomatyki okresu dorastania i dorosłości*, (155–168), Lublin: PROQURAT.

Teresiak, E., Czarnecka-Operacz, M., Jenerowicz, D. (2006). Wpływ nasilenia stanu zapalnego skóry na jakość życia rodzinnego chorych na atopowe zapalenie skóry. *Postępy Dermatologii i Alergologii*, 23, 249–257.

Tuszyńska-Bogucka, W. (2007). *Funkcjonowanie systemu rodziny z dzieckiem przewlekle chorym dermatologicznie*. Lublin: Wydawnictwo UMCS.

Wyczesany, J., Ostrowski, T.M., Lohn, Z. (2000). *Indywidualne i społeczne czynniki determinujące aktywny udział dzieci chorych w procesie leczenia*, Kraków: Oficyna Wydawnicza Impuls.

Izabella Januszewska, Stanisława Steuden
The John Paul II Catholic University of Lublin
Institute of Psychology

STYLES OF COPING WITH NEGATIVE EMOTIONS AND STRESS IN PATIENTS WITH HYPERTENSION

Abstract

The goal of the study was to answer the question: which and what are the specific styles of coping with negative emotions (anger, anxiety, sadness) and stress used by healthy individuals as compared to those suffering from hypertension?

The study involved 203 people from 50 to 65 years of age, where the clinical group consisted of 100 hospitalized patients suffering from hypertension and a control group of 103 healthy individuals. The study was carried out by using:

(1) The Questionnaire on Emotion Regulation (FEEL) and

(2) The Coping Orientations to Problems Experienced Scale (COPE).

It has been shown that in experiencing negative emotions and stress, non-adaptive styles and strategies for regulating negative emotions are characteristic of people with hypertension (resignation, withdrawal, self-humiliation, perseveration, $F = 7.44$, $p = 0.0001$), explaining 15.9% of the total variability of the results.

Using the method of cluster analysis on the distributions of results from both groups, six styles of coping with negative emotions and stress were identified: (1) defensive, (2) masochistic, (3) activist, (4) mildly defensive, (5) constructive and (6) confrontational ($F = 40.10$, $p = 0.0001$), showing in detail ($\chi^2 = 33.01$, $df = 5$, $p = 0.0001$) that styles 2 and 4 are more characteristic of the group of people with hypertension, whereas styles 3, 5 and 6 of healthy people. It should be noted that there is a convergence between the results obtained in this study and the research findings recently quoted in literature that cardiac symptoms associated with type "D" personalities as described by J. Denollet are characterized by a high frequency and intensity experiencing negative emotions and social inhibition demonstrated by the tendency to inhibit the expression of emotions, thoughts and behaviours.

Key words: negative emotions, stress, hypertension, coping styles, resilience

Introduction

Circulatory system diseases constitute the main cause of mortality in the world (12.8%)[1]. One in three adults has high blood pressure – a state which causes about half of all deaths, from stroke and heart diseases[2]. In prevention and treatment of cardiovascular diseases, great attention has been paid to the role of psychological and psychosocial factors. Frequent and long-term experiencing of strong negative emotions and stress, during exposure to factors that threaten psychological well-being, is particularly observable in cardiac patients, which may lead to these diseases. Taking into account that some part of the population maintain good mental and somatic health, the concept of resilience should be noted. This is defined as a dynamic process that reflects relatively good adaptation despite the threats or traumatic experiences faced by an individual (Craig et al., 2003; Sameroff et al., 2006). The essence of resilience is the ability to maintain positive emotional states and appropriate distancing from negative emotional states, which lead to physical and mental welfare. Therefore, in a clinical analysis, it is important to understand which coping styles are used by healthy people and cardiac patients in difficult situations.

R. Lazaurs – a classic on the psychological theory of stress – explains the concept of stress as "a relationship between the person and the environment that is appraised by the person as taxing or exceeding his or her resources and endangering his or her well-being" (Lazarus, 1984, by: Janowski, Steuden et al., 2009, p. 109). Due to the nature of stress, there are two concepts in studies concerning the effects of stress on the cardiovascular system: *acute stress*, which causes specific reactions, such as cardiac contractile dysfunction, myocardial ischemia, contraction of blood vessels (Rozansky et al., 1999); and *chronic stress*, which causes protracted internal tension that weakens the functioning of the cardiovascular system, as well as leading an unhealthy lifestyle (Kiecolt-Glaser, Glaser, 1999) characterized by: work overload, excessive requirements, and job dissatisfaction (e.g. Allison et al., 1995; Kalimo et al., 2000; Kubzansky et al., 1997).

A close relationship between stress and *emotions* must be mentioned here, defined by D. Dolinski as a "subjective mental state that initiates a priority for the related activity program. It is usually accompanied by somatic changes and facial, pantomime and behaviour expressions" (Dolinski, 2000, p. 322). In a stressful situation, besides the occurrence of positive emotions (in the case of dealing with the problem), there are also negative ones, such as anger, anxiety or sadness. A person has to deal with these emotions (apart from the existing stressful situation). During an experience, these levels may be confused, since we tend to identify our state of emergency and uncertainty, for example before

[1] http://www.who.int/mediacentre/factsheets/fs310/en/index.html (2013).
[2] http://www.who.int/mediacentre/news/releases/2012/world_health_statistics_20120516/en/index.html (2013).

an exam – either as fear, anxiety or stress. Therefore, many researchers regard negative emotions as symptoms or components of stress (cf. Histon, Burton, 1997, 1998; Hobfoll, 1998, 2006; Steuden, Kurtyka-Chałas, 2009, p. 130). On the theoretical level, it is difficult to distinguish these processes – the experience of stress and negative emotions – because of the similarity of physiological mechanisms (LeDoux, 2000). Scherer attempted to resolve this phenomenon and, in his opinion, emotions that are rather transient states may be turned into the state of stress in a situation when the factors that cause them are not resolved, or when a person does not have the possibility to reformulate them. According to this concept, stress is prolonged and becomes "the unresolved emotion." As a result, we encounter various forms of stress, such as stress-anger or stress-anxiety (Scherer, 1985 by: Łosiak, 2007, p. 27).

Coping with stress, according to R. Lazarus and S. Folkman (1984), is defined as "cognitive and behavioral efforts to manage specific external and/or internal demands that are appraised as taxing or exceeding the person's resources." Two general coping strategies have been distinguished: problem-oriented strategies are efforts to actively do something to alleviate stressful circumstances, whereas emotion-oriented strategies involve efforts to regulate the emotional consequences of stressful or potentially stressful events (cf. Januszewska, 2009a; Ogińska-Bulik, 2009). Grob, Smolenski (2005) described adaptive emotion regulation strategies which, in the case of the experienced problems, engage mental energy to attempt to solve a problem rather than to avoid confrontation with it. It is also often directed at external objects than on the "self." The maladaptive emotion regulation strategies engage psychic energy to suppress or avoid confrontation with the experienced problems, rather than to solve them. It also seems that it is addressed to the "self" instead of on external objects; it is also often against the "self" (by: Januszewska, 2009b).

The use of a specific style of coping with difficulties by a particular person is influenced by psychological and psychosocial factors. Many studies have focused on identifying these factors in the etiology and prognosis of cardiovascular diseases. Taking into account their historical background, initially, in the 70's of the twentieth century, they were applied to Type A behaviour. This term was coined by cardiologists Meyer Friedman and Ray Rosenman. People who manifested such behaviour were characterized as *impatient, manifesting hostility and willingness to compete and the constant struggle to achieve their objectives* (often vaguely defined) (Friedman, Rosenman, 1974, cf. Wrześniewski, 2000). The reason that type A behaviour began to be an area of interest was that these people, in comparison to others, experienced heart attacks two to three times as often (Plotnik, Kouyoumdjian, 2011, p. 495). Next, at the end of the 90's of the twentieth century, a new definition of Type A behaviour was created associated with *hostility and anger* as its main components. Studies showed that people manifesting these characteristics are three times more likely to have a heart attack, and people who quickly react with anger under stress had a five times

172

higher risk of developing precocious heart disease (Smith, 2003). Researchers concluded that a large increase in physiological arousal is observed in individuals who either always externalize anger/hostility or always suppress it, which has a harmful effect on a person's heart and health (Finney, 2002).

Currently, it is assumed that people who are at risk of cardiovascular system diseases may manifest a type D personality, which is associated with *chronic worrying, negative emotions and social inhibition.* This concept was introduced in 1996 by Johan Denollet (Denollet et al., 1996; cf. Hemingway, Marmot, 1999). This type of personality is present in the general population from 13% to 32.5%, whereas in cardiac patients from 26% to 53% (Aquarius et al., 2005; Denollet, 2005; Pedersen, Denollet, 2004; Kupper et al., 2007). The Type D personality is associated with increased cortisol reactivity to stress and, consequently, an increased risk of acquiring cardiac diseases (Aquarius et al., 2005; Conraads et al., 2006; Denollet, 2005; Denollet et al., 1995; Pedersen, Denollet, 2004; Kupper et al., 2007). Research conducted by Ogińska-Bulik (2009) among patients with hypertension showed a significantly higher intensity of their emotions and that they are also more likely to suppress them.

Despite the fact that the studies support the relationship between personality type D and health problems, it should be remembered that research on Type A behaviour also had a strong beginning. The Type D personality is a relatively new concept; therefore, carrying out more research is required in order to further demonstrate its impact on health (Miller, 2005).

Studies on the behaviour of Types A and D show that certain personality traits, such as anger/hostility and negative emotional/social inhibition, may increase the risk of cardiac disease. This means that the process of treatment of diseases of this type should not only include drug therapy, but also work on behaviour in order to decrease the level of negative traits (Merz et al., 2002).

Methodology

The research question and hypotheses

The data concerning the experience of negative emotions and stress in the etiology of hypertension clearly indicate a strong relationship between these phenomena, but their definition is still not clear and precise. Therefore, the goal of this paper is to take a step further in exploring the problem and obtaining more evidence in order to answer the question: *Is there a relationship and what is the relationship between styles of coping with negative emotions and stress in healthy individuals and those with hypertension?*

The research problem will be explained by reviewing the following research hypotheses:

H_1. People with hypertension, as compared to healthy people, are more likely to use maladaptive coping styles with negative emotions.

H_2. People with hypertension, as compared with healthy people, more often use emotion-focused strategies than problem-focused strategies.

Research methods

The Questionnaire on Emotion Regulation (*FEEL*) authored by A. Grob and C. Smolenski (2005). The translation from German into Polish and adaptation was prepared by E. Januszewska (2009a, 2009b) and A. Januszewski (2009). The *FEEL* questionnaire consists of 90 items which investigate coping strategies with basic negative emotions experienced: anger, anxiety, and sadness. For each of these emotions, there are 30 statements that relate to the 15 emotion regulation strategies (by: Januszewska, 2009b). The questionnaire in the Polish adaptation uses 23 indicators of emotion regulation. The following are the scaled summary results for both the emotions (anger, fear, sadness) individually as well as total values for all the emotions together. For the so-called diverse strategies: 1–7 (adaptive emotion regulation strategies: Problem-oriented action, Distraction, Mood enhancement, Acceptance, Forgetting, Cognitive problem solving, Re-evaluation, 8–12 (maladaptive emotion regulation strategies: Resignation, Aggressive action, Withdrawal, Self-devaluation, Perseveration) and 13–15 (other emotion regulation strategies: Social support, Externalizing, Emotional control) the raw score for each scale is calculated as the sum of the resulting answers to six items – two for aspects of anger, fear and sadness. For the so-called generalized strategies: adaptive 16–18 (for anger, fear and sadness) and maladaptive 20–22 (for anger, fear and sadness) each of the three results is the sum of points obtained in response to items characterizing each of the three emotions in controlled aspects (adaptive/maladaptive emotion regulation strategies). The two other scales (19 and 23) are the most generalized emotion regulation strategies: adaptive (1–7) and maladaptive (8–12), which are constituted by the sum of items for anger, fear and sadness.

In order to give a brief description of psychometric qualities it is worth noting that the factor analysis on a Swiss sample (N = 780) (using principal components with Varimax rotation declared by two factors: the first explains 33% and the other 17.7% of the variability of results) showed that the first factor consisted of 1–7 emotion regulation strategies, and the second of 8–12. Accordingly, the factor loadings are in the range (0.65–0.81) and (0.46–0.74; 0.36 – the lowest load demonstrated for aggressive behavior) (Grob, Smolenski, 2005).

Similar results were obtained in the study of a Polish sample (N = 430). The first factor explains 30%, the other 21.1% of the variability of results, where the first factor consisted of 1–7 emotion regulation strategies and the second factor of 8–12. Accordingly, the factor loadings were in the range (0.54–0.78) and (0.47–0.84), and that of aggressive behavior was 0.55 which is significantly higher than in the Swiss sample. The range of α-Cronbach was from 0.58 to 0.92 (Januszewska, 2009b) showing that the different scales measure psychological constructs consistently and accurately.

The Coping Orientations to Problems Experienced Scale (*COPE*), whose authors are: Ch. Carver, M. Scheier and J. Weintraub (1989). This tool is used to study the way in which people react to stress and is related to the R. Lazarus transactional model of stress (Lazarus and Folkman, 1984) and a model of behavioural self-regulation (Scheier and Carver, 1988). The inventory contains 60 items, which are put into 15 strategies (4 in each strategy) (see Juczyński, Ogińska-Bulik, 2009).

Participants

The study was conducted on cardiac patients in a hospital from november 2011 to february 2012. They were selected randomly and came from various regions in Poland. The study involved 203 people aged 50 to 65. The clinical group consisted of 100 patients during hypertension rehabilitation. The second (control) group consisted of 103 healthy individuals who were selected according to the criterion 1:1 (socio-demographic similarity) in relation to the clinical group.

Results

The statistical procedures used in the study (one-way and multivariate analysis of variance) are based on the group paradigm in two ways: (1) as a result of the specificity of the participants belonging to the group of patients with hypertension *vs.* healthy people, (2) as a result of the *ex post facto* (*EPF*) procedure, in which the entire test sample ($N = 203$) was subjected to the typology procedure, expecting to identify the impact of structural types (coping styles with negative emotions), significantly (*F*-test, $p \leq 0.05$) more characteristic of "patients" in comparison to "healthy" people. It is worth noting that most of the important research problems in the field of social and educational sciences are not suitable for solving experimentally, whereas many of them can be answered through controlled research of the *ex post facto* (Kerlinger, 1964 for: Brzeziński, 1996, p. 451).

According to this paradigm, a researcher attempts to identify unknown to them independent variables (affiliation of the respondents to the style), which gives the dependent variable specific values for the studied population. Since unknown independent variables (sometimes occurring a long time ago) influenced a given dependent variable, therefore, the only thing that can be done is an attempt to identify them by *ex post* analysis (Kerlinger, 1964 for: Brzeziński,

1996, p. 432). According to this paradigm, the independent variables are styles for coping with negative emotions (anger, anxiety, sadness), which in this study were controlled by the *FEEL* questionnaire scales.

Hypertension and coping with negative emotions

The contents of this section are a comparison between patients and healthy people in adaptive and maladaptive fields generalized by negative emotions strategies. The term "generalized" covers two aspects of psychological constructs, such as: adaptability/maladaptability and similarity of responses within each of the constructs, regardless of whether the emotional state is related to the experience of anger, anxiety or sadness.

Table 1. Analysis of variance: comparison of average scores in FEEL scales: adaptive (16–18) and maladaptive (20–22) generalized strategies of negative emotions: anger, anxiety, sadness in groups of patients and healthy individuals. Sample: N = 203 (patients with hypertension: Men n_1 = 53, Women n_2 = 47; healthy individuals: Men n_3 = 49, Women n_4 = 54)

Groups → ↓ Generalized negative emotions strategies:				**Patients** (group 1) **M + F** (n_1 = 100)	**Healthy** (group 2) **M + F** (n_2 = 103)	The significance of dif. bet. groups (1–2)		eta² × 100 = value in %
						F	p =	
Adaptive	anger	16	M	5.81	5.36	2.58	0.110	1.3%
			s	2.10	1.90			
	anxiety	17	M	5.63	5.35	0.96	0.327	0.5%
			s	2.10	1.97			
	sadness	18	M	5.53	5.58	0.04	0.848	0.0%
			s	2.14	1.75			
Maladaptive	anger	20	M	5.97	5.16	9.17	0.003	4.4%
			s	1.81	2.02			
	anxiety	21	M	5.91	5.17	6.97	0.009	3.4%
			s	1.98	1.99			
	sadness	22	M	5.89	5.08	9.46	0.002	4.5%
			s	1.91	1.86			
MANOVA (scales 16–18, gr. 1–2) F = 1.83 df_1 = 3 df_2 = 199 p = 0.142								2.7%
MANOVA (scales 20–22, gr. 1–2) F = 3.90 df_1 = 3 df_2 = 199 p = 0.010								5.6%

176

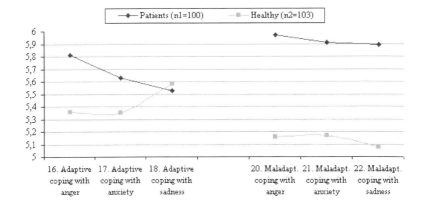

Figure 1. Comparison of average scores on the FEEL scales: adaptive (16–18) and maladaptive (20–22) generalized strategies of negative emotions: anger, anxiety, sadness in groups of patients and healthy individuals

In reviewing the data presented in Table 1 and in Figure 1, it can be concluded that the independent variable (health/hypertension) has a significant impact on the distribution of the dependent variables in terms of the maladaptive emotion regulation strategy from experienced anger, anxiety and sadness. There was no such dependence in relation to adaptive strategies[3]. The score of the multivariate analysis of the variance test (MANOVA: $F = 3.90$, $p = 0.010$) indicates that patients cope worse than healthy individuals, with the appeasement of negative emotional states caused by the experience of anger, anxiety and sadness. This is confirmed by a more detailed degree of analysis. A generalized non-adaptive strategy for coping with sadness (ANOVA: $F = 9.46$, $p = 0.002$) is much more typical for patients than healthy people. These patients much more often (and with much higher intensity) initiate maladaptive regulation strategies to calm the experienced sadness. Similar regularity has also been shown in relation to both maladaptive coping with anger (ANOVA: $F = 9.17$, $p = 0.003$) and anxiety (ANOVA: $F = 6.97$, $p = 0.009$). This means that patients with hypertension experienced anger (which is a response to loss of control during activities and efforts as a consequence of frustration) and anxiety – and these are clearly appeased with maladaptive emotion regulation strategies.

When analyzing the second ternary set, which is an argument of a generalized adaptive emotion regulation strategies construct, it can be observed that

---

[3] In Polish adaptation of the *FEEL* questionnaire used confirmatory factor analysis studies to show that the correlation between the primary construct for adaptation scales (16–18) and construct for maladaptation scales (20–21) of emotion regulation strategies of anger, anxiety and sadness is not statistically significant ($r = -0.06$, $p > 0.05$). This means that the two constructs are sovereign in relation to each other, i.e., if we see clear signs of maladaptive coping with anger in someone's behaviour, we cannot conclude that the person does not use or have a repertoire of adaptive coping with that emotion (or vice versa) (see Januszewska, 2009b).

it has no significant correlation with the independent variable. The results of the multivariate analysis of the variance test (MANOVA: $F = 1.83$, $p = 0.142$) did not reach statistical significance ($p \leq 0.05$), indicating that the problem of "health/hypertension" does not affect the whole construct of adaptive emotion regulation strategies and, derived from it, behaviour related to the regulation of negative emotional states caused by the experience of anger, anxiety and sadness. Concerning three dependent variables (anger, anxiety, and sadness) – in terms of generalized adaptive emotion regulation strategies – the two groups are very similar to each other.

Hypertension and styles of coping with negative emotions

In going from the level of generalized negative emotions strategies to the level of differentiated strategies and then to the styles of coping with negative emotions – we initially performed a multivariate analysis of variance on sets of variables that are differentiated indicators of adaptive and maladaptive negative emotion regulation strategies. The first set includes: (1) Problem-oriented action, (2) Distraction, (3) Mood Enhancement, (4) Acceptance, (5) Forgetting (6), Cognitive problem solving, (7) Re-evaluation. The study of the relationship between affiliation to patient groups *vs.* healthy individuals and the distribution of results in the set of dependent variables showed no significant correlation ($F = 1.54$, $p = 0.157$; $eta^2 \times 100 = 5.2\%$). The differentiated maladaptive indicators are: (8) Resignation, (9) Aggressive action, (10) Withdrawal (11) Self-devaluation, (12) Perseveration. In this case, the connection is very clear ($F = 7.44$, $p = 0.0001$; $eta^2 \times 100 = 15.9\%$). Summarizing, it has been shown that the fact of belonging to a group of patients or healthy individuals is significantly associated with the variability of results among maladaptive negative emotion regulation strategies at both levels: generalized and differentiated indicators. Such evidence was not proved in terms of adaptive strategies indicators.

Taking into account the above-mentioned fact, from the matrix derived from the entire test sample ($N = 203$), which is the set of variables representing the maladaptive strategies (8–12), a group of people representing different structural styles of coping with negative emotions was isolated. Technically, the non-hierarchical cluster analysis algorithm was used here, according to the procedure determined by the k-means. The optimal was a 6-clustered solution.

Table 2. Belonging to groups representing various styles of coping with negative emotions and the criterion of "patient" or "healthy." The significance of differences in the distributions was marked with the "z" test. Lower values of significant difference (p ≤ 0.05)* is 2

Styles→	Style 1	Style 2	Style 3	Style 4	Style 5	Style 6	
	defensive $(n_1 = 20)$	masochist $(n_2 = 45)$	activist $(n_3 = 33)$	mild. def. $(n_4 = 36)$	constru. $(n_5 = 33)$	confront. $(n_6 = 36)$	(N = 203)
	9.8%	22.2%	16.3%	17.7%	16.3%	17.7%	100%
"patient"	60.0%	64.4%	33.3%	77.8%	21.2%	36.1%	49.3%
"healthy"	40.0%	35.6%	66.7%	22.2%	78.8%	63.9%	50.7%
"z" test	1.0	2.3*	2.0*	3.8*	3.5*	1.7•	

In order to verify *ex post* if belonging to one of the six clusters is related to the fact of participants belonging to their original assignment, the "patient" (n_1 = 100) and "healthy" (n_2 = 103) – Chi^2 test was performed, whose result (33.01, df = 5, p = 0.0001) confirms the hypothetical assumption that there are groups of people (clusters) more typical of either the "patients" or the "healthy." The extension of this general observation with the "z" test allowed showing which of the six groups representing the styles of coping with negative emotions is more characteristic for the "patients" and the "healthy" groups. The following coping styles are typical for people suffering from hypertension: mildly defensive (4) and masochistic (2), and for healthy people: activist, (3) and in particular constructive (5). A tendency ($p \leq 0.1$), with a loaded probability error less than 10% can be noted that healthy people more often use a confrontational style (6). It should also be added that a defensive style (1) is characteristic of the first mentioned observation, with 9.8% of the whole sample, indicating that 60% of the group consists of patients and 40% of healthy individuals. Although this regularity is not statistically significant, it is similar to the one that describes the fourth style, giving the group of "patients" a special mark – more frequent and stronger use of defensive forms of resolving tensions caused by the presence of negative emotions as well as their consequences.

A more detailed description of the above dependences is presented in Table 3, showing the average value in the range of psychological variables (differentiated emotion regulation strategies), which formed the basis of the identification of the independent variable (the *ex post facto* procedure), i.e. coping with negative emotions represented by groups of people isolated by cluster analysis.

The structure of maladaptive emotion regulation strategies represented by five scales at 47.7% is explained by the fact of specificity resulting from the classification of people into one of the six styles of coping with emotions (MANOVA: F = 40.10, p = 0.0001). The interaction test (styles x groups) did not show a significant association (MANOVA: F = 1.02, p = 0.444) with the distribution of the dependent traits.

Table 3. Analysis of variance: A comparison of average scores on scales of differentiated maladaptive regulation strategies with negative emotions (8–12) FEEL for groups of people isolated by cluster analysis (k-means) representing 6 styles of coping with negative emotions (anger + anxiety + sadness). Sample: N = 203 (patients with hypertension: Men n_1 = 53, Women n_2 = 47; healthy individuals: Men n_3 = 49, Women n_4 = 54)

Styles → ↓ Scales of differentiated maladaptive regulation strategies with negative emotions through:		Groups of people representing various coping styles with negative emotions and the averages in maladaptive scales of emotion regulation strategies						The significance of differences between styles (1–6)			eta^2 x 100 = value in %
		(Style 1) defen. (n_1 = 20)	(Style 2) masoch. (n_2 = 45)	(Style 3) activ. (n_3 = 33)	(Style 4) mild. de. (n_4 = 36)	(Style 5) constru. (n_5 = 33)	(Style 6) confron. (n_6 = 36)	df_1 = 5; df_2 = 197		Games-Howell Test (α = 0,05)	
								F	p =		
Resignation 8	M	8.45	5.00	4.09	6.94	3.30	6.36	70.32	0.0001	[1–2,3,4,5,6][2–3,4,5,6] [3–4,6][4–5][5–6]	64.1%
	s	1.05	1.38	1.13	1.29	1.10	1.13				
Aggressive action 9	M	6.60	4.29	5.79	4.92	4.12	8.00	46.94	0.0001	[1–2,4,5,6][2–3,6] [3–4,5,6][4–6][5–6]	54.4%
	s	1.47	1.59	0.99	1.23	1.32	1.04				
Withdrawal 10	M	8.60	5.47	4.79	6.64	3.06	5.75	59.55	0.0001	[1–2,3,4,5,6][2–4,5][3–4,5,6][4–5,6][5–6]	60.2%
	s	0.88	1.49	0.96	1.20	1.22	1.32				
Self-devaluation 11	M	7.55	7.64	3.82	5.53	4.88	4.11	62.37	0.0001	[1–3,4,5,6][2–3,4,5,6] [3–4,5][4–6]	61.3%
	s	1.42	1.11	1.31	1.19	1.27	1.14				
Perseveration 12	M	7.60	5.20	3.85	6.86	3.85	6.56	39.52	0.0001	[1–2,3,5][2–3,4,5,6] [3–4,6][4–5][5–6]	50.1%
	s	1.35	1.46	1.18	1.31	1.50	1.44				
MANOVA (scales 8–12, styles 1–6) F = 40.10 df_1 = 25 df_2 = 718 p = 0.0001											47.7%
MANOVA (scales 8–12, styles 1–6 x groups 1–2) F = 1.02 df_1 = 75 df_2 = 842 p = 0.444											8.0%

It is worth noting that the styles of coping with negative emotions, as described below, were separated on the basis of the maladaptive construct and its scales. However, not all of them should be regarded as non-adaptive. They differ not in the value of maladaptiveness, but also in respect to the quality resulting from the structure of different styles. Generally, activist and constructive coping (3 and 5) can certainly be considered as a form of adaptive regulation of negative emotions, whereas defensive and mildly defensive coping (1, 4) can be regarded as rather non-adaptive; masochistic coping style (2) – due to the typicality of directing negative emotions into oneself, this may have signs of destructive auto-aggression; confrontational coping (6) reveals the typicality of negative emotions by acting out the aggression against other people, i.e. within the nearest social environment.

Style 1: **Defensive** coping. Under the influence of events that cause negative emotions in people representing a defensive coping style, a feeling of their own powerlessness and lack of control occurs (Resignation ↑) with a very clear tendency of passive tolerance of this unpleasant state, and a lack of willingness to engage in mental and behavioural improvement in both the mental state and the situation that caused it (Withdrawal ↑). As a result, these people do not collect personal experiences which might be beneficial, if only a problematic situation is solved creatively. All of this makes it impossible to overcome the barriers of a vicious circle, and a person with a feeling of progressive loss of influence on the events and directing their failures onto themselves experiences feelings of guilt and shame or depressive reaction (Re-evaluation ↑). Due to these factors and a high propensity to maintain and refresh negative emotions for a long time, almost obsessively (Perseveration ↑), these people, in order to reduce the experienced unpleasant emotional state, despite its short-term effects, might become aggressive towards people and/or items that are not necessarily related to a problematic situation (Aggressive action ↑).

This style represents 9.8% of the sample, and outlining this tendency is more typical in the group of patients with hypertension (60%) than healthy people (40%).

Style 2: **Masochistic** coping. The experienced permanent and high level of guilt, shame and pessimism generates in these people an interpretation of the roots of failures and frustrations especially in themselves (Self-devaluation ↑). Therefore, negative, often quite complex emotions appear, which are not directed externally (Aggressive action ↓) but internally, against themselves.

This style represents 22.2% of the sample, and is significantly ($p \leq 0.05$) more dominant in patients with hypertension (64.4%) than in healthy individuals (35.6%).

Style 3: **Activist** coping. The representatives of this style, influenced by events that cause negative emotions, do not lose faith in themselves and their abilities, treating all the failures and frustrations as triggered by external factors and possible to overcome. These people might have a slightly inflated self-image (Self-devaluation ↓) and they do not maintain negative emotions for long, but rather take on activity aimed at solving the problem (Perseveration ↓). Such an approach towards themselves permits them to feel that they have personal power to influence events, so they not only exhibit significant activity in their behaviour (Resignation ↓) but do not give up (Withdrawal ↓) taking action, which consequently leads to collecting many new personal experiences and generating a feeling of well-being.

This style represents 16.3% of the sample and is significantly ($p \leq 0.05$) more dominant in healthy (66.7%) than in the hypertensive group of people (33.3%).

Style 4: **Mildly defensive** coping. Similarly to the first of presented above, it is a passive tolerance of an unpleasant emotional state (Withdrawal ↑), a feeling of their own powerlessness and lack of control over events (Resignation ↑) and a strong tendency to maintain and refresh negative emotions for long, almost obsessively (Perseveration ↑). The difference between these two styles is that in the mildly defensive style of coping, structural components are not as strong as those outlined in defensive coping. It might be observed that, despite a tendency to resign, in reactions and withdrawal from life situations in which they must confront and solve problems and deal with unpleasant consequences of the experienced frustrations, they make a minimum effort to somehow relieve dystonic emotions. Also, aggressive behaviours are not generally used by these people (Aggressive action ↓). Hypothetically, this coping style may be a way of responding to their disease.

This style represents 17.7% of the sample, of which a significant portion ($p \leq 0.05$) is dominant in patients with hypertension (77.8%) as compared to healthy individuals (22.2%).

Style 5: **Constructive** coping. For these individuals, the experience of an unpleasant emotional state becomes an activator of the action (Resignation ↓), so they always take steps aimed at the real root of the problem, creatively solving it (Withdrawal ↓) adequately. Slightly lower self-esteem in a stressful situation becomes a challenge and a motivating factor to help settle the problem (Self-devaluation ↓). These people do not reveal aggression directed towards themselves or towards external objects (Aggressive action ↓) due to a constructive solution to the problem, instead of repeating it in obsessive thoughts (Perseveration ↓).

This style of coping might be regarded as a model from an empirical point of view. People who use this style represent the mature ability to cope with stress and its negative consequences and a competent, integrated ego.

This style represents 16.3% of the sample, and significantly more often ($p \leq 0.05$) dominates in healthy (78.8%) than in the hypertensive group (21.2%).

Style 6: **Confrontational** coping. It becomes particularly significant in the context of the presence of other people who may become an addressee of aggressive attacks in getting over negative emotions (Aggressive action ↑), which are also obsessively maintained by them (Perseveration ↑). In addition, these people are unable to reconcile with the experience of unpleasant emotional states, which indicates their personal weakness and weakening effect on the event. Confrontational-aggressive behaviour expressed towards people from the environment might also have their origin in selecting the propensity to resignation from solving the problem (Resignation ↑) and, related to it, low self-esteem and the accumulation of negative emotions (Self-devaluation ↓).

This style represents 17.1% of the sample, and significantly more often ($p \leq 0.05$) dominates in healthy (63.9%) than in the hypertensive group (36.1%).

Overall, the research material described above is the basis for verification of the research hypotheses (H_1) and confirms that people with hypertensive disease often use maladaptive coping styles with negative emotions (anger, anxiety, sadness).

Hypertension and coping with stress

The research material is the basis for demonstrating the relationship between the independent variables: (1) belonging to the group of patients *vs.* healthy individuals, and (2) belonging to the style of coping with negative emotions and classically understood dependent variables, which are scales of the strategies for coping with stress that are shown in Tables 4 and 5. These variables are a part of the transactional model of psychological "coping" presented by R. Lazarus and S. Folkman. Regularities that are presented here are the basis for the verification of the hypothesis that people with hypertension, as compared to healthy people, rarely use strategies which are directed at solving the problem, but often use emotion-focused strategies (H_2).

Table 4. Analysis of variance: A comparison of average results in a The Coping Orientations to Problems Experienced Scale (*COPE*) in groups of patients and healthy people. Sample: N = 203 (patients with hypertension: Men n_1 = 53, Women n_2 = 47; healthy individuals: Men n_3 = 49, Women n_4 = 54)

Groups →			Patients	Healthy	The significance of differences b. gr. (1–2)		eta² × 100
			(group 1) M + W	(group 2) M + W			= value in %
↓ Coping with stress scales:			(n_1 = 100)	(n_2 = 103)	F	p =	
Active coping	1	M	5.19	5.51	1.52	0.220	0.7%
		s	1.93	1.83			
Planning	2	M	5.37	6.09	7.25	0.008	3.5%
		s	1.75	2.04			
Seeking Instrumen. Social Support	3	M	5.28	5.90	5.83	0.017	2.8%
		s	1.76	1.91			
Seeking Emotional Social Support	4	M	5.14	5.97	8.51	0.004	4.1%
		s	1.92	2.13			

Suppression of competing activity	5	M	5.09	5.77	6.45	0.012	3.1%
		s	1.59	2.16			
Turning to religion	6	M	5.46	5.46	0.00	0.989	0.0%
		s	2.04	1.83			
Positive reinterpr. and growth	7	M	5.18	5.70	4.05	0.046	2.0%
		s	1.73	1.93			
Restraint coping	8	M	5.61	5.25	1.91	0.168	0.9%
		s	1.83	1.85			
Acceptance	9	M	5.83	5.29	4.20	0.042	2.0%
		s	1.98	1.76			
Focusing on and venting of emotions	10	M	5.17	5.86	6.38	0.012	3.1%
		s	1.83	2.07			
Denial	11	M	6.04	5.00	18.15	0.0001	8.3%
		s	1.73	1.74			
Mental Disengagement	12	M	5.80	5.76	0.02	0.878	0.0%
		s	2.11	1.86			
Behavioural disengagement	13	M	5.90	4.94	12.31	0.001	5.8%
		s	1.96	1.93			
Alcohol/drug use	14	M	6.17	5.74	4.49	0.035	2.2%
		s	1.61	1.28			
Humour	15	M	5.78	4.82	15.95	0.0001	7.4%
		s	1.71	1.73			
MANOVA (scales 1–15, gr. 1–2) F = 3.36 df_1 = 15 df_2 = 187 p = 0.0001							21.2%

A multivariate analysis of the variance test shows that the distribution of results in the set of variables that represent the stress coping strategies are highly dependent on the impact of belonging to a group of patients *vs.* healthy people (MANOVA: $F = 3.36$, $p = 0.0001$), explaining 21.2% of the variability.

There should be noted a clearly stronger frequency of coping by denying (ANOVA: $F = 18.15$, $p = 0.0001$) in patients than in healthy individuals, which is based on ignoring, avoiding and rejecting the fact that a difficult situation occurs. The result may be that patients with hypertension, as comparing to healthy individuals, might have more difficulties in being adequately involved in new events. Additionally, due to the experience of stress patients – more often than healthy people – operate with an acceptance strategy (ANOVA: $F = 4.20$, $p = 0.042$) which does not have the form of functional behaviour (expressing the acceptance of the situation and making efforts to learn how to live with it), but rather is an expression of the lack of active coping, being a consequence of their assuming a lack of personal resources and seeing the situation as irreversible. Also, a significantly higher frequency of humour as a strategy (ANOVA: $F = 15.95$, $p = 0.0001$) is used among patients, who treat a sense of humour as a temporary appeasement of unpleasant emotions, but this indicates rather avoidance behaviour than solving the root of the problem. The behavioural disengagement (ANOVA: $F = 12.31$, $p = 0.001$) strategy which to a much greater extent is used by the patients also shows the dominance of avoidance behaviour in the form of resignation of efforts to achieve the goals and their experience of helplessness. In addition, patients, more often than healthy people, are more likely to consume alcohol or other psychoactive substances (ANOVA: $F = 4.49$, $p = 0.035$) in order to temporarily calm unpleasant emotions, which indicates more frequent use of their avoidance behaviour.

On the other hand, healthy individuals in a stressful situation to a much greater extent not only seek emotional social support (ANOVA: $F = 8.51$, $p = 0.004$) involving the search for moral support and understanding in others, but also instrumental social support (ANOVA: $F = 5.83$, $p = 0.017$) in the form of advice, assistance or information, which indicates problem-focused solving. What is more, healthy people, as compared to patients, operate more often by planning a strategy (ANOVA: $F = 7.25$, $p = 0.008$), which means more frequently considering whether they have the resources to deal with the problem. Suppression of competing activities (ANOVA: $F = 6.45$, $p = 0.012$) is also more typical of healthy individuals, which indicates that they are more likely to avoid other activities that are not related to the problem in order to better cope with it. Healthy people, to a higher degree, focus on and vent emotions (ANOVA: $F = 6.38$, $p = 0.012$) and worry about them, which might motivate them to active behaviour, oriented towards problem solving. In the case of coping with stress, healthy individuals more often experience positive reinterpretation and growth (ANOVA: $F = 4.05$, $p = 0.046$), which on the one hand concerns concentrating on emotions, but on the other, by noticing the event's core values, it stimulates the source of personal development and constitutes evidence of a problem-focused strategy.

Styles of coping with negative emotions and coping with stress

Strategies for coping with stress, represented by fifteen scales at 14.9% are explained by the specificity resulting from the classification of people into one of the six styles of coping with negative emotions (MANOVA: $F = 2.16$, $p = 0.0001$). The interaction test (style x belonging to a group of patients/healthy people) did not show a significant association with the distribution of the dependent variables (MANOVA: $F = 1.04$, $p = 0.327$).

Table 5. Analysis of variance: A comparison of average results in The Coping Orientations to Problems Experienced Scale (*COPE*) for groups of people separated by the cluster analysis (k-means) representing 6 styles of coping with negative emotions (anger + anxiety + sadness). Sample: N = 203 (patients with hypertension: Men n_1 = 53, Women n_2 = 47; healthy individuals: Men n_3 = 49, Women n_4 = 54)

Styles → ↓ Coping with stress scales:			Groups of people representing various coping styles with negative emotions and the averages on *COPE* scales						The significance of differences between styles (1–6) df_1 = 5; df_2 = 197			eta^2 x 100
			(Style 1) defen. (n_1 = 20)	(Style 2) masoch. (n_2 = 45)	(Style 3) activ. (n_3 = 33)	(Style 4) mild. de. (n_4 = 36)	(Style 5) constru. (n_5 = 33)	(Style 6) confron. (n_6 = 36)	F	p =	Games-Howell Test (α = 0.05)	= values in %
Active coping	1	M	5.15	6.11	4.67	5.00	5.73	5.17	3.13	0.010	[2–3]	7.4%
		s	1.76	1.95	1.80	1.59	1.79	2.02				
Planning	2	M	5.15	5.96	6.00	5.36	6.70	5.03	3.74	0.003	[5–4.6]	8.7%
		s	1.92	1.77	2.15	1.44	1.96	1.95				
Seeking instru. soc. support	3	M	5.20	5.40	5.64	5.39	6.03	5.83	0.85	0.518		2.1%
		s	2.04	1.71	1.87	1.76	1.86	2.04				
Seeking emotion. social support	4	M	5.15	5.11	5.73	5.39	5.58	6.36	1.79	0.116	[2–6]	4.4%
		s	2.58	1.61	2.23	2.03	2.11	1.99				
Suppression of competing activit.	5	M	5.40	5.51	4.67	5.17	7.15	4.75	8.80	0.0001	[5–1.2.3.4.6]	18.2%
		s	1.98	1.91	1.51	1.40	2.11	1.61				
Turning to religion	6	M	5.20	5.44	5.36	5.69	5.70	5.25	0.37	0.866		0.9%
		s	2.31	2.20	1.48	1.80	1.65	2.16				
Positive reinterpr. and growth	7	M	5.25	5.93	5.18	4.94	6.24	4.94	3.25	0.008		7.6%
		s	1.80	1.72	1.94	1.64	2.03	1.69				
Restraint coping	8	M	6.40	5.64	4.91	5.64	5.18	5.11	2.25	0.051		5.4%
		s	1.90	1.89	2.13	1.42	1.93	1.62				
Acceptance	9	M	6.55	5.84	4.97	5.61	5.33	5.33	2.22	0.054	[1–3]	5.3%
		s	1.70	2.07	2.11	1.59	1.88	1.64				
Focusing on and venting of emo.	10	M	5.80	5.04	5.55	5.44	5.67	5.89	0.89	0.488		2.2%
		s	1.80	1.60	2.28	2.14	2.23	1.83				
Denial	11	M	6.25	5.69	4.85	5.92	4.39	6.11	5.95	0.0001	[5–1.2.4.6]	13.1%
		s	1.97	1.58	1.94	1.59	1.58	1.72				
Mental disengagement	12	M	6.20	5.47	5.45	6.03	5.82	5.94	0.75	0.591		1.9%
		s	2.29	1.83	2.03	2.02	1.91	1.99				
Behavioural disengagement	13	M	7.05	5.22	4.91	5.94	4.48	5.53	5.74	0.0001	[1–2.3.5] [4–5]	12.7%
		s	2.19	2.01	1.86	1.67	1.62	2.02				
Alcohol/drug use	14	M	6.05	5.80	5.94	6.14	5.42	6.39	1.76	0.122	[5–6]	4.3%
		s	1.61	1.46	1.52	1.48	0.94	1.64				
Humour	15	M	5.45	5.18	4.67	5.44	5.27	5.78	1.48	0.196		3.6%
		s	1.76	1.67	1.69	1.54	1.83	2.11				
MANOVA (scales 1–15, coping styles 1–6) F = 2.16 df_1 = 75 df_2 = 881 p = 0.0001												14.9%
MANOVA (scales 1–15, coping styles 1–6 x groups 1–2) F = 1.04 df_1 = 225 df_2 = 1792 p = 0.327												8.4%

These source psychological descriptions made on the basis of distributions of the results shown in Table 3 will be complemented by the contents of the results shown in Table 5. In this general way, coping with emotions will be linked with stress.

Style 1: **Defensive** coping. In situations causing the occurrence of negative emotions in people representing a defensive coping style, there is a high sense of helplessness, which results in resigning from their efforts to achieve goals and passively tolerating the presence of an unpleasant state (Behavioural disengagement ↑). Several subsequent, clearly avoiding strategies used by these individuals are: acceptance, which is an expression of the lack of active coping as a consequence of a belief about the lack of one's personal resources and the occurring situation as irreversible (Acceptance ↑); avoiding thinking about the consequences of the event by engaging in other activities (Mental disengagement ↑); a tendency to use alcohol or drugs to alleviate temporarily unpleasant emotions (Alcohol/drug use ↑); and even to deny or reject the situation (Denial ↑). A high passiveness in behaviour can also be explained by these people in their anticipating the right moment to solve the problem (Restraint coping ↑).

Style 2: **Masochistic** coping. Comparing the results in the distribution of the dependent variables, it was shown that people operating in a masochistic coping style (as compared with other groups) are characterized by special activity aimed at removing or reducing the stressor or its consequences (Active coping ↑).

Style 3: **Activist** coping. The representatives of this way of coping, due to their high self-confidence, do not allow the thought of not resolving the problem. They treat a difficulty which occurred very seriously (Humor ↓) and do not accept it in any of its aspects, nor do they intend to simply get used to it (Acceptance ↓) or to devote much attention to it either (Denial ↓). They never resign from efforts to achieve the objectives (Behavioural disengagement ↓), but their actions may be premature and hasty (Restraint coping ↓). Therefore, their actions are not necessarily intended to really eliminate or reduce the stressor (Active coping ↓), but might be directed at totally different aspects, unrelated with the problem (Suppression of competing activities↓).

Style 4: **Mildly defensive** coping. People operating in a mildly defensive coping style, as well as those who use a defensive one, manifest passivity in their behaviour when experiencing difficult situations, although it should be noted that symptoms can be recognized to a slightly lower degree. These people tend to avoid thinking about the consequences of the event by engaging in other activities (Mental disengagement ↑), and use alcohol or drugs to alleviate temporarily unpleasant emotions (Alcohol/drug use ↑). The passivity among these people can be explained by the fact that they have difficulties in perceiving in the event values for personal development and in finding the positive aspects that could motivate them to undertake activities (Positive reinterpretation and growth ↓).

Style 5: **Constructive** coping. There is a mature ability to cope with stress among this group of people, the result of their being pro-active and highly concentrated on solving the source of the problem. Experiencing difficult situations, these people, in order to make the most constructive use of their energy, first of all direct it towards adequately planning and considering the most effective strategies to cope with the stressor (Planning ↑), at the same time avoiding unnecessary interventions which are not related to the problem (Suppression of competing activities↑). Besides decisions they themselves make, they also appreciate the sharing of experiences with others, which constitutes one source of knowledge for them (Seeking Instrumental Social Support ↑). It should also be noted that, while struggling with the problem, they do not deny the situation as an escape from it (Denial ↓), but simply treat it as a challenge that they want to wrestle with. They perceive superior values in this action, which are a valuable source of strength for them (Positive reinterpretation and growth ↑), so that they do not easily resign from achieving their objectives (Behavioural disengagement ↓).

Style 6: **Confrontational** coping. These people, overloaded with many negative emotions, do not consider a solution to the problem as their primary goal, but instead use highly emotion-focused strategies. The solution to the problem, in fact illusory, is temporarily achieved by a feeling of security and support from others, which is why they seek it in difficult situations (Seeking Emotional Social Support ↑). These people are so emotionally overwhelmed that they do not see value in an event they should fight for (Positive reinterpretation and growth ↓). Lack of ability to cope with stress and experienced dystonic states are associated with: operating with avoidance behaviour, drug/alcohol use in order to alleviate temporarily unpleasant emotions (Alcohol/drug use ↑); denial, the rejection of the problematic situation (Denial ↑); engaging in other activities that are not related to the problem (Suppression of competing activity ↓). As a result, these behaviours do not solve the problem, but additionally enhance the feeling of lack of control, which generates a further source of unpleasant emotions.

Summary and general conclusions

The purpose of this study was to attempt to define the relationship between styles of coping with negative emotions and stress in patients with hypertension. The empirical material presented above, its formal analysis and substantive interpretation constitutes the basis for the formulation of conclusions whose content is used to verify the research hypotheses.

The contents of the first hypothesis (H_1) are verified positively. A multivariate analysis of the variance test shows that the distribution of results in the set of variables that represent the differentiated maladaptive regulation strategies with negative emotions is highly dependent on the impact of belonging to a group of patients/healthy people (MANOVA: $F = 7.44$, $p = 0.0001$), explaining 15.9% of the total variance of the results. There is an observable convergence between the results obtained in this study and the research findings quoted in the literature that cardiac symptoms and associated with them D-type behaviour is characterized by a high frequency and intensity of the experience of anger/hostility, and a tendency to irritability, withdrawal, and social inhibition evident in the inhibition to express emotions, thoughts and behaviours in contact with others (see Pelle et al., 2010).

In further steps of the analyses, the structure of maladaptive emotion regulation strategies represented by five of the above mentioned scales allowed for the separation of six styles of coping with emotions (MANOVA: $F = 40.10$, $p = 0.0001$; $eta^2 = 47.7\%$): (1) defensive, (2) masochistic, (3) activist, (4) mildly defensive, (5) constructive, (6) confrontational (see Table 1, Figure 1). A more detailed analysis has shown that ($Chi^2 = 33.01$, $df = 5$, $p = 0.0001$) styles 2 and 4 are more characteristic of a group of people suffering from hypertension, while styles 3, 5 and 6 are more typical of healthy people (see Table 1).

Moreover, it has been shown that it was not the variables which belong to the adaptive strategies that significantly differentiate comparing groups (in this case they are similar to each other), but the psychological variables belonging to the maladaptive strategies that have a significant part in explaining the analyzed problem (see Table 1, Figure 1).

The second hypothesis (H_2) was also positively verified with obtained evidence ($COPE$) (see Tables 4 and 5). A multivariate analysis of the variance test showed that the distribution of the results in the set of variables that represent the strategies for coping with stress is highly dependent on the impact of belonging to a group of patients/healthy people (MANOVA: $F = 3.36$, $p = 0.0001$), explaining a total of 21.2% of the variability of the results. Similar results showing that people with hypertension are highly focused on their emotions were also obtained in other studies (see Ariff; Suthahar, 2011; Sher, 2009; Sheridan, Radmacher, 1998).

The significantly higher results obtained by a group of "patients" on the following scales: (9) Acceptance (11) Denial, (13) Behavioural disengagement, (14) Alcohol/drug use, (15) Humour – show more intense use of emotional forms of coping with defensive avoiding-escaping behaviour.

The results suggest that people with hypertension to a much lower degree than healthy people operate in a cooperative style, so that they might receive support from people in their social environment. The arguments here are the significantly lower results obtained on the scales: (3) Seeking instrumental social support, (4) Seeking Emotional social support and (10) Focusing on and venting of emotions.

On the level of comparisons between groups of people representing the structural styles (1–6) of coping with negative emotions, the most specific observation can be clearly related to people representing a constructive coping style (5), of which one-fourth refers to people with hypertension and three-fourths to healthy individuals. Other differences shown in the presented table might be due to the influence of other independent variables (neither hypertension nor lack of it), which are not considered in this study.

In conclusion, worthy of consideration are the interpretative hypotheses explaining the origin of psychological constructs, the styles of coping with negative emotions and stress with the presented regularities in this article, which on the one hand imply a picture of health in bio-psycho-social aspects, and on the other, are a source of knowledge about the content and forms of counselling and health-oriented prevention. The essence of resilience is to generate and intentionally use the adaptive coping styles appropriate to the situation rather than those maladaptive strategies correlated to aggravated somatic, psychic and social health. Work on the development of resilience and adaptive coping styles for difficult situations can be defined as a developmental process by which people acquire the ability to use internal and external resources in order to achieve an adequate level of adaptation despite past or currently occurring stressors.

References

Allison, T., Williams, D., Miller, T. (1995). Medical and Economic Costs of Psychological Distress in Patients with Coronary Artery Disease. *Mayo Clinic Proceedings*, 70, 734–742.

Ariff, F., Suthahar, A. (2011). Coping styles and lifestyle factors among hypertensive and non-hypertensive subjects. Singapore Medical Journal. *Singapore Medical Journal*, 52, 1, 29–34.

Aquarius, A., Denollet, J., Hamming, J., De Vries, J. (2005). Role of disease status and Type D personality in outcomes in patients with peripheral arterial disease. *American Journal of Cardiology*, 96, 996–1001.

Carver, C., Scheier, M., Weintraub, J. (1989). Assessing coping strategies: A theoretically based approach. *Journal of Personality and Social Psychology*, 56, 267–283.

Conraads, V., Denollet, J., De Clerck, L., Stevens, W., Bridts, C., Vrints, C. (2006). Type D personality is associated with increased levels of tumour necrosis factor (TNF)-alpha and TNF-alpha receptors in chronic heart failure. *International Journal of Cardiology*, 113, 34–38.

Craig, A., Bond, L., Burns, J., Vella-Brodrick, D., Sawyer, S. (2003). Adolescent resilience: a concept analysis. *Journal of Adolescence*, 26, 1–11.

Denollet, J. (2005). DS14: Standard assessment of negative affectivity, social inhibition, and Type D personality. *Psychosomatic Medicine*. 67, 89–97.

Denollet, J., Sys, S., Stroobant, N., Rombouts, H., Gillebert, T., Brutsaert, D. (1996). Personality as independent predictor of long term mortality in patients with coronary heart disease. *Lancet*, 347, 8999, 417–421.

Denollet, J., Sys, S., Brutsaert, D. (1995). Personality and mortality after myocardial infarction. *Psychosomatic Medicine*, 57, 582–591.

190

Doliński, D. (2000). *Mechanizmy wzbudzania emocji*. [W:] J. Strelau (red.). *Psychologia. Podręcznik akademicki*, T. 2. (321–322). Gdańsk: Gdańskie Wydawnictwo Psychologiczne.

Finney, M., Stoney, C., Engebretson, T. (2002). Hostility and anger expression in African-American and European American men is associated with cardiovascular and lipid reactivity. *Psychophysiology*, 39, 340–349.

Friedman, M., Rosenman, R. (1974). *Type A Behaviour and Your Heart*. New York: Knopf.

Grob, A., Smolenski, C. (2005). *FEEL-KJ. Fragebogen zur Erhebung der Emotionsregulation. Manual*. Bern: Verlag Hans Huber, Hogrefe AG.

Hemingway, H., Marmot, M. (1999). Evidence based cardiology: psychosocial factors in the aetiology and prognosis of coronary heart disease. Systematic review of prospective cohort studies. *BMJ*, 318, 1460–1467.

Histon, J., Burton, R. (1997). A psychophysiological model of psystress causation and response applied to the workplace. *Journal of Psychophysiology*, 11, 200–217.

Hobfoll, S. (1998). Stress, Culture and Community. *The Psychology and Philosophy of Stress*. New York: Plenum.

Hobfoll, S. (2006). *Stres, kultura i społeczność. Psychologia i fizjologia stresu*. Gdańsk: Gdańskie Wydawnictwo Psychologiczne.

Janowski, K., Steuden, S., Kuryłowicz, J., Nieśpiałkowska-Steuden, M. (2009). *The disease – related appraisals scale: A tool to measure subjective perception of the disease situation*. [W:] K. Janowski, S. Steuden, *Biopsychosocial Aspects of Health and Disease*, Lublin: CPPP, 108–125.

Januszewska, E. (2009a). *Uwarunkowania strategii regulacji emocji złości, lęku i smutku u młodzieży*. [W:] L. Szewczyk, E. Talik (red.). *Wybrane zagadnienia z psychologii klinicznej i osobowości. Psychologia kliniczna nastolatka*. Lublin: Towarzystwo Naukowe Katolickiego Uniwersytetu Lubelskiego, 235–258.

Januszewska, E. (2009b). *Konfirmacyjne modele strategii regulacji emocji negatywnych. Badania eksploracyjne młodzieży*. [W:] L. Szewczyk, E. Talik (red.). *Wybrane zagadnienia z psychologii klinicznej i osobowości. Psychologia kliniczna nastolatka*. Lublin: Towarzystwo Naukowe Katolickiego Uniwersytetu Lubelskiego, 259–296.

Januszewski, A. (2009). *Strategie i style regulacji emocji negatywnych*. [W:] L. Szewczyk, E. Talik (red.). *Wybrane zagadnienia z psychologii klinicznej i osobowości. Psychologia kliniczna nastolatka*. Lublin: Towarzystwo Naukowe Katolickiego Uniwersytetu Lubelskiego, 297–337.

Juczyński, Z., Ogińska-Bulik, N. (2009). *Wielowymiarowy Inwentarz do Pomiaru Radzenia Sobie ze Stresem – COPE*. [W:] *Narzędzia Pomiaru Stresu i Radzenia Sobie ze Stresem*. Warszawa: Pracownia Testów Psychologicznych, 23–44.

Kalimo, R., Tenkanen, L., Haermae, M., Poppius, E., Heinsalmi, (2000). Job stress and sleep disorders: findings from the Helsinki Heart Study. *Stress Medicine*, 16, 65–75.

Kiecolt-Glaser, J., Glaser, J. (1999). Chronic Stress and Mortality Among Older Adults. *JAMA*, 282, 23, 2259–2260.

Kubzansky, L., Kawachi, I., Spireo, A. (1997). Is Worrying Bad for Your Heart? A Prospective Study of Worry and Coronary Heart Disease in the Normative Aging Study. *Circulation*, 95(4), 818–824.

Kupper, N., Denollet, J. (2007). Type D Personality as a Prognostic Factor in Heart Disease: Assessment and Mediating Mechanisms. *Journal of Personality Assessment*, 89, 3, 265–276.

Lazarus, R., Folkman, S. (1984). *Stress, appraisal and coping*. New York: Springer.

LeDoux, J. (2000). *Mózg emocjonalny. Tajemnicze podstawy życia emocjonalnego*. Poznań: Media Rodzina.

Łosiak, W. (2007). *Psychologia emocji*. Warszawa: Wydawnictwa Akademickie i Profesjonalne.

Merz, B., Dwyer, J., Nordstrom, C., Walton, K., Salerno, J., Schneider, R. (2002). Psychosocial stress and cardiovascular disease: pathophysiological links. *Behav. Med.*, 27, 4, 141–147.

Miller, A. (2005). *The social psychology of good and evil*. New York, NY, US: Guilford Press.

Ogińska-Bulik, N. (2009). *Osobowość typu D: teoria i badania*. Łódź: Wydawnictwo WSHE.

Pedersen, S., Denollet, J. (2004). Validity of the Type D personality construct in Danish post-MI patients and healthy controls. *Journal of Psychosomatic Research*, 57, 265–272.

Pelle, A., Broek, K., Szabo, B., Kupper, N. (2010). The relationship between Type D personality and chronic heart failure is not founded by disease severity as assessed by BNP. *International Journal of Cardiology*, 145, 1, 82–83.

Plotnik, R., Kouyoumdjian, H. (2011). *Introduction to psychology*, CA: Wadsworth Publishing, 480–507.

Rozansky, A., Blumenthal, J., Kaplan, J. (1999). Impact of Psychological Factors on the Pathogenesis of Cardiovascular Disease and Implications for Therapy. *Circulation*, 99, 16, 2192–2217.

Sameroff, A., Rosenblum, K. (2006). Psychosocial Constraints on the Development of Resilience. *Annals of the New York Academy of Sciences*, 1094, 116–124.

Scheier, M., Carver, C. (1988). A Model of Behavioral Self-Regulation: Translating Intention into Action, *Advances in Experimental Social Psychology: Social Psychological Studies of the Self*, 21, 303–346.

Sher, L. (2009). *Psychological Factors and Cardiovascular Disorders: The Role of Stress and Psychosocial Influence*. New York: Nova Science Publisher.

Sheridan, C., Radmacher, S. (1998). *Psychologia zdrowia. Wyzwanie dla biomedycznego modelu zdrowia*. Warszawa: Instytut Psychologii Zdrowia.

Smith, W., Salovey, Rothman, J. (Ed.) (2003). *Hostility and health: Current status of a psychosomatic hypothesis. Social psychology of health. Key readings in social psychology*. New York: Psychology Press, 325–341.

Steuden, S., Kurtyka-Chałas, J. (2009). *Dynamika procesu przeżywania straty związanej ze śmiercią współmałżonka*. [W:] S. Steuden, S. Tucholska (red.). *Psychologiczne aspekty doświadczania żałoby*. Lublin: Wydawnictwo Katolickiego Uniwersytetu Lubelskiego, 123–144.

Wrześniewski, K. (2000). *Style a strategie radzenia sobie ze stresem. Problemy pomiaru*. [W:] I. Heszen-Niejodek, Z. Ratajczak (red.). *Człowiek w sytuacji stresu*. Katowice: Wydawnictwo Uniwersytetu Śląskiego, 44–63.

Krzysztof Gerc
Jagiellonian University
The Institute of Applied Psychology

Marta Jurek
Jesuit University Ignatianum in Cracow

FAMILY LIFE DIMENSIONS AND SELF-ASSESSMENT OF ADOLESCENTS AND YOUNG ADULTS USING PSYCHOACTIVE SUBSTANCES – THE COMPARATIVE STUDY

Abstract

This article, the theoretic principles of which have been based on the concept of protective factors of J.D. Hawkins' and Circle Model of D.H. Olson, considers the problem of relation between family life dimensions and bonds in family systems and using psychoactive substances by adolescents and young adults. The experimental group consisted of 32 individuals between the ages of 17 to 25 who have used psychoactive substances and the control group consisted of 34 years randomly chosen group at the comparable ages. The objection of the studies have been, among other things, to verify the hypotheses suggesting the relation between negative experience of communication and bonds in family (family functioning worse in dimension of *cohesion* and *flexibility*) and using psychoactive substances.

In the studies have been used: the biographic questionnaire developed by the authors of the article, Family Relationships Questionnaire (FRQ) by Mieczysław Plopa, Family Assessment Scale (FAS) and Multiple Self-Assessment Questionnaire MSEI by O'Brein and Epstein. The results of the analysis prove conclusively that individuals from experimental group receive lower outcomes in the following dimensions of their families functioning: *cohesion*, *flexibility*, *rigidity*, while higher ones described as *lack of bonding*. No statistically significant or direct relation has been proved between the quality of communication and using the psychoactive substances.

Key words: self-assessment, context of using psychoactive substances, family life

Introduction

The characteristic of communication process in perspective of current theoretic conclusions

The notion of communication belongs to arising controversy issues. The controversy refers not only to culture differences when interpreting the process of communication itself but the controversy also results from different research approaches creating specific and of their own perspectives for interpretation of communication. Although some researchers (see Pankiewicz, 2007) consider in practice only three approaches: mechanistic, psychological and systematic as significant believes in theory and practice in the field of communication research we can destinguish as much as seven theories of communication: sociopsychological, cybernetic, retoric, semiotic, evaluative, sociocultural and phenomenological (Griffin, 2003). Yet it is observed that despite the approach represented by the individual researcher, the assumed desired effect of communication is optimal, adequate and effective.

The notion means most generally (Kubisa-Ślipko, 2004, p. 36) *getting communicated, conveying the thoughts, giving the news.* Suggested by different researchers, definitions and frames of the process of communication are determined by the paradigm represented by their authors. S. Dylak [1997] distinguishes three basic ones. The first one is the paradigm of transmission of knowledge. In that paradigm communication is understood as transmission of a specific message from the sender to recipient throughout a certain channel existing in a specific environment. In that model communication is only of contents character. The second paradigm, called interactive one, highlights appearing thanks to transmitted message and mutual understanding interactions. The third – transactional one – also highlights the interactions but understands them as a technique of getting understanding by a series of mutual negotiations.

Noticing and appreciating so called "body language" contributed to distinguishing non-verbal communication understood as "the way in which people communicate intentionally or unintentionally without words" (Aronson, Wilson, Akert, 1997, p. 173) and recognising "mimic expressions, tone of voice, gestures, body posture and movements, touch and looking as the indicators of non-verbal communication" [p. 173]. The verbal communication has been distinguished separately and as its opposition and its meaning has been limited to "getting communicated by the signs of language" (Pilch, 2003, p. 707). R.J. Sternberg (2001, p. 248) connected and tried to balance those two ways of communication assuming that "communication is an exchange of thoughts and feelings which may or may not contain language because relies also on non-verbal forms such as gestures and looks etc."

The fact of common use of the notion of communication (see Skorupka, 1988, p. 69) makes some researchers to distinguish the concept of "interpersonal communication." Such distinction has been made by W. Szewczuk (1979, p. 120), according to whom "interpersonal communication is transmission of a message between the sender and the recipient (…) who should be affected by it in a certain way (result in a change of his/her actions, attitude, believes)." S. Frydrychowicz also uses a term of interpersonal communication and underlies rather relation and emotion in communication. He claims it being a process in which "a sender gives his/her emotional attitude towards not only the content of the message but also to the recipient. During communication the relation between the sender and the recipient is constantly defined an redefined" (Frydrychowicz, 2003, p. 105). Similarly R. Griffin claims communication being "a bilateral constant process in which we use verbal and non-verbal messages in cooperation with the other person to create and modify images aroused in minds of the participants of the process of communication" (Griffin, 2003, p. 74). Interesting and very precise understanding of communication represents P. Winterhoff-Spurk to whom communication is

> such a process in which two or more participants tuned into interaction and mutually affecting each other on the base of similar definition of situation and similar set of signs using systematically variable verbal and non-verbal means of communication transfer the message to partner/partners of communication so that what is thought would be understood and what is wanted would be done (Winterhoff-Spurk, 2007, p. 10).

Such an understanding of communication, because of its precision and adequacy towards those facets of communication which are being assessed in Olson's Circle model described in a further part of the article, has been accepted in the study.

Communication and D.H. Olson's Circle Model and theory of systems

It should be highlighted that communication as a process is a part of numerous other models. One of them is a D.H. Olson's Circle Model (Margasiński, 2006; 2010; 2011) that is founded on three family life dimensions: "cohesion, flexibility, communication. Cohesion is understood as the emotional bond which the pair and individual family members give to each other" (Olson, Gorall, 2003, p. 3). The model allows to describe cohesion at one of five levels: not bounded/disconnected, slightly bounded, bounded, strongly bounded and tangled. Only those central, except two extreme levels allow for maintaining the balance in the family system and at the same time keeping the feeling of independence and nearness by its members.

The second dimension – "flexibility means the number of changes taking place in leadership, changeability of rules and roles taken in a relationship" (the above, p. 6) That dimension is being assessed at following levels: stiff/not flexible, slightly flexible, flexible, very flexible and chaotic. Just the same as it is for the first dimension, the extreme levels are considered as not being beneficial for functioning of the system while the others allow to keeping the homeostasis in the system.

The third dimension – communication – plays an adaptive role for the whole family system within both above defined dimensions. Playing such an important role in the system is possible thanks to such components of communication as "ability of listening and speaking, self-disclosure, clarity, following the subject, respect and mindfulness" (the above, p. 7). Such named facets of communication remarkably determine the ability of empathy, exchange of experiences, discussion on the topic, respecting and appreciating the emotional climate of the talk. It should be also highlighted that examined in the D.H. Olson's Circle Model dimensions result from systems the theory.

Analysis of the own research

Research methodology

The study, being a part of a bigger research project, was aimed at testing whether there is a difference in perceived interpersonal family communication between using psychoactive substances research group and a control group not using them. It has been also tried to decide whether there is a relationship between self-esteem and specific communication style and specific relationships in families of the examined individuals. The research group consisted of 66 individuals aged between 17 and 25 years (the average age was 21 and three months). 32 of them (the average age 21 years and 8 months old) has used illegal psychoactive substances some time at their lifetime and belonged to the research group and 34 belonged to control group (the average age 20 years and 4 months old). The majority of the examined individuals have been the graduates of high school (8 individuals in research group and 9 in control group have been at general education lyceum, the others were the students of higher education or working). All the examined individuals originated from Lesser Poland (the majority, that is 14 in research and 16 in control group gave Kraków (Cracow) as the place of living). Anonymous in the form study was conducted from October 2011 to June 2012. The following research methods have been used: the author's questionnaire developed for purpose of the research and aimed at gaining information on using psychoactive substances by the examined individuals, *Family Assessment Scale* (FAS) adapted by Andrzej Margasiński, Mieczysław Plopa's *Family Relationship Questionnaire* (FRQ), O'Brein's and Epstein's *Multiple Self-assessment Questionnaire.*

The notion of "psychoactive substances" most often is identified as "drugs" (see Sierosławski, Zieliński, 2000; Cabalski, 2009) or "addictive substances" (see Gacek, 2000). In literature most often it is referred to "changing mental functioning substances" (Carson, Butcher, Mineka, 2006, p. 552) or rather more precisely "medicinal or non-medicinal substances all having ability of modifying moods and behavior" (Piotrowski, 1992, p. 163). The latter definition seems to be universal that way that it allows to take into account also currently being legal substances but used in order to get intoxicated as well as chemical compounds in some other products but affecting the functioning in a way similar to drugs (for instance so called "designer drugs").

Using research questions based on the available literature, the following hypotheses have been made:

Hypothesis 1.1 The research group assesses their family communication as worse than the control group.

Hypothesis 1.2 Individuals who assess their family interpersonal communication as worse take illegal psychoactive substances more often.

Those hypotheses are grounded on the assumptions of R. Jessor's theory that classified as psychosocial risk factors among others: modeling of the environment and availability of the support coming from the environment (Jessor, 1987; Jesor et al., 1995; Jessor, 1998; Costa, Jessor, Turbin, 2007).

The results of longitudinal research taken among adolescent boys by R. Loeber and his colleagues (1998) have shown that besides the poor communication in the family, low school achievement, attention deficit hyperactivity disorder, insufficient parental control may also have been related to using psychoactive substances and behavioral disorders, aggression, depression, shyness and withdrawal.

In literature there is belief that communication makes an inspiration for normally functioning family in terms of flexibility and cohesion that consequently condition well adapting to dynamic changes of the environmental conditions (Westermeyer, 1998; Olson, Gorall, 2003).

Hypothesis 2. The research group assesses their families as worse functioning in respect of flexibility and cohesion than the control group. That hypotheses is grounded on, among others, the J.D. Hawkins's (1992; 2005) and in Poland K. Okulicz-Kozaryn's and K. Bobrowski's (2009) research according to which one of the most strongly connected with lessening risk of problematic behaviour factor are the positive bonds with one's parents. Those bonds can be described on the level of flexibility and cohesion.

Hypothesis 3. The individuals of research group show lower self-esteem than the control group's individuals. Similarly, that hypotheses is grounded on Richard Jessor's (1998) and W.B. Hansen's (1992; 1993; 2004) theory which defines individual or social vulnerability to display such behaviour and low self-esteem may turn out being the predetermining factor (see. Costa, Jessor, Turbin, 2007).

Hypothesis 4. The low self-esteem correlates with the outcomes received on scales of communication. While grounding that hypotheses, the observation that inadequate level of self-esteem favours non-partner style of communication (Harwas-Napierała, 2008) has been recalled.

The research outcomes – verifying the hypothesis

While verifying hypothesis 1.1 and 1.2, the following operationalisation has been made: the research and control group differ significantly in respect of outcomes received at *Communication* sub-scales of the FAS and FRQ questionnaires.

Student's t-test for independent groups has been used in order to test the significance of the difference between two groups, while assuming the variance being equal. The results are shown in Table 1.

Table 1. The results of the test of significance of differences between the research and control group in respect of assessment of family communication

	Statistics for groups				Test of means' equality				
	Group	N	Mean	Standard deviation	t	df	Significance (one-sided)	Means' differ- ence	Stan- dard error
Communica- tion FAS	Control	32	35,24	9,11	1,32	63	0,097	3,11	2,372
	Research	31	32,13	9,77					
Communica- tion FRQ	Control	32	28,78	6,24	1,41	63	0,072	1,90	1,694
	Research	31	26,88	6,72					

Source: own

Hypothesis 1.1 has not been proved – statistic analysis has not shown any statistically significant difference between the research and control groups' outcomes on *Communication* sub-scales of FAS and FRQ questionnaires. The research group has shown lower outcomes on both sub-scales but the difference has turned out not to be statistically significant. Negative verification of hypotheses 1.1 might be caused by a small sample.

While verifying the hypothesis 1.2, it has been decided to distinguish frequency of using the psychoactive substances at present and the amount of substances taken in individual's lifetime. In order to verify that hypotheses, the analyses of correlation has been used, because all the variables are measured on interval scales following nearly normal distribution.

Tables 2 and 3 show the outcomes of that analyses.

Table 2. Correlation coefficient between the declared by the examined individuals frequency of using substances and the outcomes received on *Communication* sub-scales of FAS and FRQ questionnaires, (N = 32)

Correlations			
		Communication FAS	Communication FRQ
How often do you take drugs?	Pearson's correlation	0,181	0,052
	significance (one-sided)	0,161	0,379
	N	31	31

Source: own

Table 3. Correlation coefficients between the declared by the examined individuals quantity of substances used at specific life periods and the outcomes received on *Communication* sub-scales of FAS and FRQ questionnaires (N = 32)

		Correlations	
		Communication FAS	Communication FRQ
Quantity of substances used at individual's lifetime	Pearson' coefficient	−0,373	−0,286
	Significane (one-sided)	**0,042**	**0,127**
Quantity of substances used during one year	Pearson' coefficient	−0,170	−0,171
	Significane (one-sided)	0,354	0,341
Quantity of substances used during last three months	Pearson' coefficient	−0,480	−0,053
	Significane (one-sided)	0,788	0,752

Source: own

Hypothesis 1.2 has been proved partially. No relation between the frequency of using psychoactive substances and perceived by the examined group quality of their family communication has been found (Table 2), but analyses has shown a small negative correlation between the quantity of substances used at one's lifetime and the outcomes on scale of communication of FAS questionnaire. The result means that the more substances individuals have experimented with at their lifetime the worse they assess their family communication abilities defined as ability of listening and following the subject, mutual respect and empathy. Should be however noticed that described dependance is rather weak and demands verification in further research.

While verifying hypothesis 2, the following operationalisation has been suggested: the research and control group differ statistically in respect of outcomes received on scales of communication of FAS questionnaire referring to such dimensions as *flexibility (Well-balanced flexibility, Stiffness, Incoherence)* and coherence (*Well-balanced coherence, Lack of bonds, Entanglement*). In order to verify hypothesis 2. Student's t-test for independent groups has been used while assuming variance being equal, with one-sided level of significance. That assumption has not been taken only for *Well-balanced coherence* variable.

A part of the differences has turned out to be statistically significant. Table 4 shows the results.

Table 4. Test of significance of difference between the research and control group in respect of outcomes on FAS questionnaire's scales measuring well-balance or lack of equality and coherence

	Statistics for groups				T-test for equality of means					
	Group	N	Mean	Standard deviation	Standard error of the mean	t	df	significance (one-sided)	Difference of means	Standard error of the difference
FAS lack of bonds	Control	32	16,33	5,42	0,94					
	Research	31	19,62	6,24	1,16	−2,19	62	0,016	−3,29	1,46
FAS stiffness	Control	32	18,42	3,98	0,69					
	Research	31	15,44	4,43	0,82	2,70	62	0,003	2,91	1,065
FAS incoherence	Control	32	16,45	5,75	1,001					
	Research	31	20,03	5,60	1,04	−2,47	62	0,007	−3,59	1,43
FAS well-balanced coherence	Control	32	27,03	4,58	0,80					
	Research	31	23,65	7,56	1,40	2,07	45	0,02	3,36	1,62
FAS well-balanced flexibility	Control	32	21,94	5,74	0,99					
	Research	31	19,41	5,42	1,01	1,69	62	0,05	2,48	1,41

Source: own

Hypothesis 2.0 has been proved. Difference between research and control group has turned out to be statistically significant. It has been found also that those examined individuals who use psychoactive substances receive lower outcomes on *Family Assessment Scale* than control group. It means that research group significantly more often perceive their families as using too usual and schematic solutions in new situations. The examined individuals assess also rules established in their families as less legible and changes in leadership as more unpredictable. Significance of difference within variable: *perceived stiffness* has also been found. The research group receive lower outcomes on subscale *stiffness* than the control group. It means that individuals perceive their families as less controlling or such ones in which leader's decisions are imposed to the other members of the family more rarely. Thus it is possible to assume with some caution that lack of clearly defined rules concerning leadership and sharing out duties as well as too much flexibility in responding to challenges might foster using psychoactive substances by adolescents and young adults.

It should also be noticed that using psychoactive substances individuals define their family relationships as less well-balanced in dimensions of intimacy and independence. It is also remarkable that individuals who use psychoactive substances statistically do not differ significantly from not using the substances individuals on outcomes on scale of *entanglement*. However, they receive lower outcomes on scale of *lack of bonding*. Thus they perceive their families as more engaging the members of the system into mutual relations and showing smaller level of independence among family members. Statistic analyses has not shown any intergroup differences for general indexes for *flexibility* and *cohesion*. The research group has received lower outcomes, but that dependance has turned out to be statistically insignificant. Because previous hypothesis have been partially confirmed, it may be assumed that the reason for that is too small number of examined individuals.

While verifying hypothesis 3, the following operationalisation has been suggested: research group receives lower results on *MSEI* questionnaire sub-scales. The hypothesis was verified by Student's t-test for independent groups while assuming variances being equal for majority of scales. Equality of variance has not been assumed for *Identity Integration*.

Table 5 shows statistically significant differences for research and control group in outcomes received on scales of MSEI.

Table 5. Statistically significant differences for research and control group in outcomes received on scales of MSEI

	Statistics for groups				T-test for eqality of means				
	Group	N	Mean	Standard deviation	Standard error of the mean	t	df	significance (one-sided)	Difference of means	Standard error of the difference
Identity integration	Control	33	32,91	8,0248	1,396	2,91	57	0,002	5,12	1,75
	Research	29	27,79	5,6969	1,058					
Moral self-esteem	Control	33	39,30	6,1516	1,071	1,80	64	0,031	3,31	1,78
	Research	29	35,97	7,7941	1,447					
Being loved	Control	33	36,18	7,4559	1,298	2,30	64	0,014	4,30	1,86
	Research	29	31,86	7,2492	1,346					
Defensive enhancement of self-esteem	Control	33	48,73	6,6298	1,154	3,08	64	0,002	6,09	2,03
	Research	29	42,62	9,1159	1,692					

Source: own

As Table 5 shows, research group individuals get lower outcomes on scales of *being loved, moral self-esteem, defensive enhancement of self-esteem, identity integration.* It means that in comparison to control group, the research group individuals may feel less acceptance and more often experience rejection from their nears. They may show slightly bigger difficulties in establishing relationships with other people and more often act against their personal believes.

While verifying hypothesis 4, the following operationalisation has been suggested: outcomes received on scales of FAS and FRQ correlate positively with the outcomes for individual scales of MSEI questionnaire.

In order to verify hypothesis 4, correlation analyses has been used.

Table 6 shows significant correlation coefficients for all self-esteem scales of MSEI and communication scales of FAS and FRQ.

Table 6. Significant correlation coefficients for individual self-esteem scales of MSEI and communication scales of FAS and FRQ

MSEI scales	Communication FRQ		Communication FAS	
	Pearson's correlation	Significance (one-sided)	Pearson's correlation	Significance (one-sided)
Vitality	0,215	0,043	0,291	0,01
Competences	0,333	0,003	0,313	0,008
Leadership capabilities	0,317	0,009	0,211	0,045
Identity integration	0,329	0,004	0,315	0,001
Physical attraction	0,268	0,017	0,360	0,001
General self-esteem	0,495	0,009	0,521	0,0003
Being loved	0,631	0,0001	0,622	0,0001
Defensive enhancement of self-esteem	0,250	0,023	0,271	0,013
Popularity	0,431	0,009	0,411	0,0005

Source: own

The research founding have provided the evidence for hypothesis 4. Its verification has shown the strong positive correlation between *communication* measured on both sub-scales and *Being loved.* It means that the higher the examined individuals assess their family communication, that is ability of listening, being empathic, respect for different opinion, the more they feel accepted and loved and maintaining close relations with other people is easier for them.

Statistic analyses has proved also moderate positive correlation between communication measured on both scales and scales *General self-esteem, Popularity.* Low positive dependence has been shown for scales: *Competences, Leadership capabilities, Identity integration, Defensive enhancement of self-esteem, Physical attraction, Vitality.* It may be expected that individuals who better assess interpersonal communication in their families, considered themselves being more competent and qualified and learn new things without any difficulties. They may show satisfaction when leading other people; they consider themselves being stronger and decisive people. Their general self-esteem is higher, so they have shown tendency of thinking about themselves in a more positive way and they depreciate their own value rarely.

Discussion of results

Although the carried out study has not proved directly clear relationship between the quality of communication in family system and using psychoactive substances, it is hard to negled indirect relations which should be scrutinised in the future research by using multiple variable correlation – regression analyses broadened with path analyses. The outcomes received in two following areas: *cohesion* and *flexibility* show indirect relation between dependable variable (*quality of communication*) and other variables distinguished in the examination that, as it has been mentioned earlier, may be regulated and are adjustable to the family needs in the process of communication of their members.

Indirect, however without doubt of high importance, affect of quality of communication in the family system has been proved by founded in the study dependence between positive assessment of the course of process of communication in the family and sense of being loved, what consequently increases family life satisfaction, helps entering and maintaining satisfying emotional bonds with other people and affects perception of one's own physical and sexual attractiveness. This observation is highly important because as the latest researches show *the need of being loved* and at the same time *readiness to love* are ones of the most important values declared by adolescents (Gerc, 2010). Besides low sense of individual's attractiveness and social competences favors using psychoactive substances. It is easily observed that using alcohol is aimed at overcoming one's shyness and initiating spontaneity in relations with the opposite sex people (Rogowska, 2009). L.S. Ham's and D.A. Hope's (2005) have shown that using psychoactive substances grows nearly proportionally with the experienced level of *social anxiety*. As early as in nineties the relation between using psychoactive substances and expectation of getting a specific social benefit, for instance lowering the tension, increase of sexual desire or enhancement of life's joy has been discovered (Aktan et al., 1997; Seto, Barbaree, 1995; Yamada et al., 1996). Later studies more and more often find connection between using psychoactive substances and higher level of aggression, using violence and even social maladjustment (Rostampour, 2000; Schubart, 2000), what was manifested with habitual choosing escape strategy when coping with stress (Borecka-Biernat, 2011).

Using psychoactive substances adolescents and young adults in comparison to individuals not taking them assessed their families as acting in a more schematic way in different problematic situations and showing specific behaviour, no matter what would be its anticipated effectiveness. It seems that some schematic way of behaviour may favour its low effectiveness, what affects not only persistence of the specific problem occurred in the family system, but often even deepens it and decreases internal locus of one's control and self-appraisal as well as decrease in general life satisfaction in individuals affected with the problem. Inaccuracy of decisions taken independently by young people is particularly painful and increases the probability of taking psychoactive substances. It is confirmed also by M. Cabalski (2009, p. 13), according to whom taking psychoactive substances "distracts from (…) hopeless struggle against everyday difficulties (…) Often taking drugs is a form of escape from troubles and one's weaknesses. In a wide spectrum of escape behaviour different ways of acting out of stress, inhibiting of anxiety or enhancing one's self-esteem occur (...) Often initiation covers failures in family or/and school life." Meanwhile K. Gerc's, B. Piasecka's and I. Sikorska's carried out among students of generally available gymnasium studies (2011) have shown that as much as 61% youth people declares the need of success. Other studies prove also that higher tendency towards taking care for one's health and avoidance of psychoactive substances are shown by those adolescents who consider themselves as their own success creators and so show statistically significantly higher level of resourcefulness (t = 3,14, p = 0,03) and self-acceptance (t = 3,11, p = 0,025) and more rarely they attribute it to favourable external factors (Gerc, Ziółkowska, Jurek, 2009).

Also interestingly, individuals using psychoactive substances more rarely have assessed their family relations as based on *nearness* and *individuality*. Instead they experienced being engaged in affairs and problems of the other and thus showed higher level of dependency more often. Those observations seem to that extend important that so far too often addicted or endangered with addiction people have been identified with social alienation or lack of strong emotional bonds within their families (Aguilar, 1992; Hansen, 1992; Hawkins, 2005). Nevertheless J. Szymańska's research conducted on a group of 365 high school students, aimed at defining the range of loneliness in youth people phenomenon, have shown that although as much as 70% adolescents admit experiencing loneliness yet almost nearly half of them (43,6%) declares that they feel it at a low level and only 4,9% at high level (Szymańska, 2009).

Research reveals also that the examined expect "sincerity, openess, being true" in a relationship with other people and creating conditions for fulfiling one's needs as well in family as in peer environment" as well in family as in peer environment [the above, p. 220]. Leading to ineffectiveness, *schematic way of acting* impedes and sometimes even quite prevents realisation of the last expectation. I should be added that theory of constructivism uses a concept of "invisible loyalties" regarding cases of some individuals and their families (Wasilewska, 2009). Those loyalties often impede young person's self-actualisation and satisfying one's needs. At the same time family obedience connected with being entangled with family relations and so-called family rituals [the above] constitutes, as K. Gerc's research (2010) has revealed – least appreciated value by endangered by addiction adolescents with high preference for independence understood in the context of taking one's own decisions.

In literature, using psychoactive substances often has been connected with unfavourable influence of the destructive peer groups in which a young person searches for authority and specific style of living (see Łapińska, Żebrowska, 1976; Vasta, Haith, Miller, 1995). Some researchers connect the phenomenon of intoxication with excessively demanding parents or high family aspirations (see Cabalski, 2009). What is more, it should be noticed that, as the results of own research, individuals taking psychoactive substances more often assessed their families to a bigger extend in comparison to control group, unpredictable in respect for leadership and less imposing on other members the rules, established by the current leader, what may result in unclear division of duties. It seems that leadership in families using psychoactive substances is not very strong and excessively controlling but in fact disturbed and expectations communicating not clear enough. Such situation does not seem to favour realisation of need of life's stabilisation declared by above half of adolescents (Gerc, Piasecka, Sikorska, 2011), neither satisfying strong need of family safety (Gerc, 2010).

Ending

The research presented in this article has been undertaken within systemic paradigm whose the main ground is a belief in circular causality and mutual feedback in family system functioning.

These results are also a part of a wider context of empirical studies conducted in recent years in Poland, which use the concept of *resilience* to the analysis and interpretation of the research results on determinants of health behavior of children and adolescents (Mazur, Tabak, 2008; Ostaszewski, 2008; Gerc, Ziółkowska, Jurek, 2009; Gerc, 2010; Borucka, Ostaszewski, 2010).

The primary objection of the study was to verify possible relationship between family functioning and particularly the quality of communication among family members and using psychoactive substances by adolescents and young adults. Making such assumption suggests, among others, David Olson's Circular Model conclusions that point at quality of communication is a vital moderator of other dimensions of family functioning.

In the summary of presented analyses of research results some conclusions can be drawn and summarised as follows:

1. No statistically significant relation has been found between quality of family communication and using psychoactive substances in examined group of adolescents and young adults. The reason for the received outcomes can be found in relatively small sample group (difficult access group) and adopted research procedure itself that is getting information about family functioning only from

one member of the system. Formulated implications refer rather to description of rather subjective perception of one's own family by particular individuals than objective verification of the reality. Yet it has been proved that using more psychoactive substances at their lifetime individuals assess their family communication as worse.

2. Needing further scrutiny as a tendency among using psychoactive substances individuals for describing their families as worse functioning (mainly for two dimensions classified by D. Olson as flexibility and cohesion) than in the control group has been found. Using psychoactive substances individuals perceive their family functioning in terms of unpredictability of behaviour, lack of clarity of rules, organisational chaos, less intense bonds. Those findings correspond with assumptions of R. Jessor's problematic behaviour.

3. It has been proved that using psychoactive substances individuals from research group show bigger difficulties in defining their own identity; they more often missed acceptance for themselves in their families and act against their own believes, striving for presenting themselves as independent and non-conformists.

4. The conducted research indicates indirectly a large number of variables which might affect young people's decisions about taking psychoactive substances and which have not been analysed in this article, neither considered in the research on which it has been based. It can be believed that relation between communication and using psychoactive substances occurs rather by their mediation. The character of that mediation should be scrutinised in further empiric research in order to establish possible direction of the relations between the variables, both causative and not causative.

References

Aguilar, T.E., Munson, W.W. (1992). Leisure education and counseling as intervention components in drug and alcohol treatment for adolescents. *Journal of Alcohol and Drug Education*, 37 (3), 23–34.

Aktan, G., Kumpfer, K.L., Turner, C. (1997). The Safe Haven program: Effectiveness of a family skills training program for substance abuse prevention with inner city African American families. *International Journal of the Addictions*, 31, 158–175.

Aronson, E., Wilson, T.D., Akert, R.M. (1997). *Psychologia społeczna. Serce i umysł*, Poznań: Zysk i S-ka Wydawnictwo.

Borecka-Biernat, D. (2011). *Temperamentalne i rodzinne determinanty obronnego sposobu radzenia sobie młodzieży gimnazjalnej w trudnych sytuacjach społecznych.* [W:] Golińska, L., Bielawska-Batorowicz, E. (red.). *Rodzina i praca w warunkach kryzysu*, (49–65). Łódź: Wydawnictwo Uniwersytetu Łódzkiego.

Borucka, A., Ostaszewski, K. (2008). Koncepcja resilience. Kluczowe pojęcia i wybrane zagadnienia. [Cz. 1]. *Medycyna Wieku Rozwojowego*, 12, 2, 587–597.

Cabalski, M. (2009). *Szkoła – Uczeń – Narkotyki. Algorytmy postępowania w przypadku stwierdzenia zażycia narkotyku przez ucznia.* Warszawa: Fundacja PEDAGOGIUM.

Carson, R.C., Butcher, J.N., Mineka, S. (2006). *Psychologia zaburzeń*, t. 1., Gdańsk: Gdańskie Wydawnictwo Psychologiczne.

Costa, F., Jessor, R., Turbin, M. (2007). College student involvement in cigarette smoking: The role of psychosocial and behavioral protection and risk, *Nicotine, Tobacco Research*, 9, 2, 213–224.

Dylak, S. (1997). *Komunikowanie się między nauczycielem a uczniem. Dwa światy – jeden język?* [W:] H. Kwiatkowska, M. Szybisz (red.). *Komunikacyjne kompetencje zawodowe nauczycieli.* „Studia Pedagogiczne", T. LXII. Warszawa: PAN.

Frydrychowicz, S. (2003). *Komunikacja interpersonalna w rodzinie a rozwój dorosłych.* [W:] Harwas-Napierała, B. (red.). *Rodzina a rozwój człowieka dorosłego*, 101–122. Poznań: Wydawnictwo Naukowe UAM.

Gacek, M. (2000). *Rozpowszechnienie substancji psychoaktywnych wśród młodzieży gimnazjalnej w Krakówie-Nowej Hucie.* [W:] *Problemy higieny*, Warszawa: Wyd. Polskie Towarzystwo Higieniczne, 69, 129–133.

Gerc, K., Ziółkowska, A., Jurek, M. (2009). *Style funkcjonowania interpersonalnego jako modyfikator wzorców zachowań prozdrowotnych młodzieży.* [W:] K. Janowski, K. Grzesiuk (red.). *Człowiek chory. Aspekty biopsychospołeczne*, t. III (20–38). Lublin: Wydawnictwo POLIHYMNIA.

Gerc, K. (2010). *Hierarchia wartości młodzieży zagrożonej uzależnieniem od środków psychoaktywnych w kontekście funkcjonowania rodziny.* [W:] G. Makiełło-Jarża (red.). *Państwo i społeczeństwo. Rodzina w przestrzeni współczesności – wybrane zagadnienia*, (88–108). Kraków: Wyd. AFM.

Gerc, K., Piasecka, B., Sikorska, I. (2011). *Uwarunkowania zachowań antyspołecznych młodzieży gimnazjalnej w kontekście funkcjonowania rodziny.* [W:] L. Golińska, E. Bielawska-Batorowicz (red.). *Rodzina i praca w warunkach kryzysu*, (31–47). Łódź: Wydawnictwo Uniwersytetu Łódzkiego.

Griffin, E. (2003). *Podstawy komunikacji społecznej*, Gdańsk: Gdańskie Wydawnictwo Psychologiczne.

Ham, L.S., Hope, D.A. (2005). Incorporating social anxiety into a model of college student problematic drinking. *Addictive Behaviors*, 30, 127–150.

Hansen, W.B. (1992). School – Based substance abuse prevention; a review of the state of the art in curriculum 1980–1990. *Health Education Research*, 7/3, 403–430.

Hansen, W., Rose, L., Dryfoos, J. (1993). Casual factors, Interventions and policy considerations in school-based substance abuse prevention. *Report submitted to Office of Technology Assessment United States Congress*, Washington: D.C.

Hansen, D.T. (2004). O rozumieniu uczniów, *Kwartalnik Pedagogiczny*, 1–2 (191–192), 43–60.

Harwas-Napierała, B. (2008). *Komunikacja interpersonalna w rodzinie*, Poznań: Wydawnictwo Naukowe UAM.

Hawkins, J., Catalano, R., Miller, J. (1992). Risk and protective factors for alcohol and other drug problems in adolescence and early adulthood: Implications for substance abuse prevention. *Psychol. Bull.*, 112, 64–105.

Hawkins, J.D. (2005). Science, social work, prevention: Finding the intersection. Aaron Rosen Lecture presented at 2005 Annual Meeting of Society for Social Work Research, *Social Work Research*, Miami: FL.

Jessor, R. (1987). Problem-behavior theory, psychosocial development, and adolescent problem drinking. *Brit. J. Addiction*, 82, 331–342.

208

Jessor, R., Van Den Bos, J., Vanderryn, J., Costa, F., Turbin, M. (1995). Protective factors in adolescent problem behavior: moderator effects and developmental change. *Develop. Psychology*, 31, 923–933.

Jessor, R. (1998). *New perspectives on adolescent risk behaviour*. [W:] R. Jessor (red.). *New perspectives on adolescent risk behavior*, (1–10). Cambridge: University Press.

Kubisa-Ślipko, A. (2004). *Słownik wyrazów obcych*, Wałbrzych: Wydawnictwo ANEKS.

Loeber, R., Farrington, D.P., Stouthamer-Loeber, M., Van Kammen, W.B. (1998). *Multiple risk factors for multiproblem boys: Co-occurrence of delinquency, substance use, attention deficit, conduct problems, physic al aggression, covert behavior, depressed mood, and shy/withdrawn behavior.* [In:] R. Jessor (Ed.). *New Perspective on Adolescents Risk Behavior*. (90–149). Cambridge: Cambridge University Press.

Łapińska, R., Żebrowska, M. (1976). *Wiek dorastania*. [W:] M. Żebrowska (red.). *Psychologia rozwojowa dzieci i młodzieży*, (664–796). Warszawa: Wydawnictwo Naukowe PWN.

Margasiński, A. (2006). Rodzina w Modelu Kołowym i FACES IV D.H. Olsona. *Nowiny Psychologiczne*, 4, 69–89.

Margasiński, A. (2010). *Rodzina alkoholowa w terapii z uzależnionym w leczeniu*. Kraków: Impuls.

Margasiński, A. (2011). *Model Kołowy i FACES jako narzędzie badania rodziny. Historia, rozwój i zastosowanie*. Częstochowa: Wyd. AJD.

Mazur, J., Tabak, I. (2008*). Koncepcja resilience. Od teorii do badań empirycznych.* [W:] J. Mazur (red.). *Czynniki chroniące młodzież 15-letnią przed podejmowaniem zachowań ryzykownych*. Warszawa: Raport z badań HBSC.

Okulicz-Kozaryn, K., Bobrowski, K.(2009). *Czynniki ryzyka, czynniki chroniące i indeksy tych czynników w badaniach nad zachowaniami problemowymi nastolatków*, online: http://www.ncbi.nlm.nih.gov/pmc/articles/PMC2671849.

Olson, D., Gorall, D. (2003). *Circumplex of marital and family systems*. [In:] F. Walsh (Ed.). *Norlam Family Processes*. New York: Guilford Press.

Ostaszewski, K. (2008), *Czynniki ryzyka i czynniki chroniące w zachowaniach ryzykownych dzieci i młodzieży*. [W:] J. Mazur (red.). *Czynniki chroniące młodzież 15-letnią przed podejmowaniem zachowań ryzykownych*. Warszawa: Raport z badań HBSC 2006.

Pankiewicz, M. (2007). *Style komunikacji a preferencje wartości uczniów zdolnych*. [W:] P. Francuz, W. Otrębski (red.). *Studia z psychologii w KUL*, t. XIV, 39–56. Lublin: Wydawnictwo Katolickiego Uniwersytetu Lubelskiego.

Pilch, T. (2003). *Encyklopedia pedagogiczna XXI wieku*, t. II. Warszawa: Wydawnictwo Akademickie ŻAK.

Piotrowski, A. (1992). *Uzależnienie od alkoholu i innych związków psychoaktywnych*. [W:] Bilikiewicz, A., Strzyżewski, W. (red.). *Psychiatria*, 163–178. Warszawa: Państwowy Zakład Wydawnictw Lekarskich,.

Rogowska, A. (2009). *Studencki wzór picia alkoholu*. [W:] K. Janowski, M. Artymiak (red.). *Człowiek chory. Aspekty biopsychospołeczne*, t. IV (555–567). Lublin: Wydawnictwo POLIHYMNIA.

Rostampour, P. (2000). Schüler als Täter, Opfer Und Unbeteiligte-Veränderung der Rollen im sozialen Und biographischen Kontext, *Psychosozial*, 23 (79), 17–27.

Schubart, W. (2000). *Gewaltprävention in Schule und Jugendhilfe: Theoretische Grundlagen, Empirische Ergebnisse, Praxismodelle*. Neuwied: Luchterhand Verlag.

Seto, M.C., Barbaree, H.E. (1995). The role of alcohol in sexual aggression. *Psychol. Rev.*, 15(6), 545–566.

Sierosławski, J., Zieliński, A. (2000). *Używanie narkotyków przez młodzież. Rozmiary i trendy zjawiska.* [W:] E. Kolarzyk (red.). *Problemy higieny.* Warszawa: Polskie Towarzystwo Higieniczne, 69, 124–128.

Skorupka, S. (1988). *Słownik wyrazów bliskoznacznych,* Warszawa: Wiedza Powszechna.

Sternberg, R.J. (2001). *Psychologia poznawcza,* Warszawa: Wydawnictwa Szkolne i Pedagogiczne.

Szewczuk, W. (1979). *Słownik psychologiczny,* Warszawa: Wiedza Powszechna.

Szymańska, J. (2009). *Kultura szkoły – jej znaczenie dla doświadczania poczucia osamotnienia przez dorastającą młodzież.* [W:] E. Augustyniak (red.). *Kultura organizacyjna szkoły* (217–225). Kraków: Uczelniane Wydawnictwa Naukowo-Dydaktyczne AGH.

Vasta, R., Haith, M., M., Miller, S.A. (1995). *Psychologia dziecka,* Warszawa: Wydawnictwa Szkolne i Pedagogiczne.

Wasilewska, M. (2009). *Siła rodzinnej tradycji.* [W:] B. Gulla, M. Duda (red.). *Silna rodzina* (48–59). Kraków: Wydawnictwo św. Stanisława.

Westermeyer, J. (1998). *Historical – social context od psychoactive substancje disorders.* [W:] R.J. Frances, S.I. Miller (Eds.). *Clinial Textbook Clinical Textbook of Addictive Disorders,* 2nd ed., (14–32). New York: Guilford Press.

Winterhoff-Spurk, P. (2007). *Psychologia mediów,* Kraków: Wydawnictwo WAM.

Yamada, T., Kendix, M., Yamada, T. (1996*).* The impact of alcohol consumption and marijuana use on high school graduation. *Health Econ,* 5, 77–92.

LIST OF AUTHORS

Tadeusz Marian Ostrowski, Ph.D., Associate Professor at the Jagiellonian University in Cracow, the Head of the Developmental and Health Psychology Department of this University's Institute of Applied Psychology, a 2nd degree of specialisation in adults clinical psychology holder. The area of interest: clinical health psychology, organizational psychology and existential psychology. The main topics of investigation: the function of the meaning of life in rehabilitation after recovery from myocardial infarction and in the treatment of cancer, resilience in the existential context, defence mechanisms in ischemic heart disease, occupational health – psychological mechanisms, especially those reducing the negative consequences of organization-related stress.
Contact: tadeusz.marian.ostrowski@uj.edu.pl

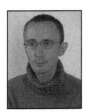

Konrad Banicki, Ph.D., is both a psychologist and a philosopher, a faculty member at the Jagiellonian University in Cracow (Institute of Applied Psychology). The areas of his interdisciplinary research include philosophy of medicine, ancient and contemporary philosophical therapy, individual differences (personality and character) as well as the various aspects of happiness and the good life.
Contact: konrad.banicki@uj.edu.pl

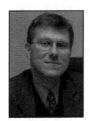

Krzysztof Gerc, Ph.D., Assistant Professor at the Developmental and Health Psychology Department, Institute of Applied Psychology, Jagiellonian University, Cracow, Poland.
His scientific interests and publications refer to: mental development of disabled people in their lifespan and the issues of supporting the development of child and young people who show developmental deficits. He deals also with the issues of culture of organization, its effect and meaning in the process of management in education and health care in the wider context of rehabilitation and educational psychology.
Contact: krzysztof.gerc@uj.edu.pl

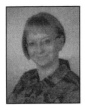

Urszula Tokarska, Ph.D., Head of The Supporting Human Development Psychological Unit, Department of Psychology, Pedagogical University of Cracow, Poland. The Unit have been created under the auspices of prof. Philip Zimbardo inside the formal structure of our Department. Main field of its interest is connected with psychological strategies of supporting human development on the different stages of life, especially via the literacy means. Author of above 30 scientific publications and 20 practical programs based on narrative and biographical approaches, one of them is the autobiographical narrative game "In Eighty Stories Around the Human Life." In preparation the book titled: "The Wheel of Life. Narrative Forms of Supporting Human Development on Every Stage of Life Course."
Contact: urszula@tokarska.pl

Iwona Sikorska, Ph.D., Assistant Professor at the Developmental and Health Psychology Department, Institute of Applied Psychology, Jagiellonian University, Cracow, Poland.
Research on resilience in children and young people including: promotion of life skills, coping with stress, adaptation to transitional life stages. A child therapist (CBT).
Scientific interests: developmental psychopathology, resilience, post-traumatic growth, philosophical anthropology.
Contact: i.sikorska@uj.edu.pl

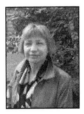

Bogusława Piasecka, Ph.D., Assistant Professor at the Institute of Applied Psychology, Faculty of Management and Social Communication, Jagiellonian University. She is a certified psychotherapist of Polish Psychological Association. She leads couples and family psychotherapy in Kraków Therapy Centre and trainings in systemic family therapy in Center for Psychotherapy and Systemic Training.
Contact: boguslawa.piasecka@uj.edu.pl

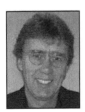

Klaus Fröhlich-Gildhoff is Professor of Developmental and Clinical Psychology at the Protestant University of Applied Sciences (EH) in Freiburg, Germany. He is as well working as psychotherapist and as supervisor for psychotherapists.
Director of the Centre for Research in Childhood and Adolescence at the EH with research projects in Early Childhood Education, Youth Welfare and Psychotherapy with children and adolescents, Head of the MA-Course "Early Childhood Education and Care," Member of the Jury of the German Prevention Award. Main topics and interests in research: promotion of mental health and resilience in early childhood (institutions) and prevention and intervention in violent behaviour.
Contact: froehlich-gildhoff@eh-freiburg.de

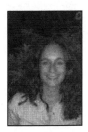

Maike Rönnau-Böse, Prof. Dr., born in 1978, is full-time professor of child education at the Protestant University of Applied Sciences (EH) in Freiburg, Germany. Her research work focuses on early childhood education, especially on resilience promotion. Furthermore, she is a trained person-centered play therapist (akt) and person-centered counselor (GwG).
Contact: roennau-boese@eh-freiburg.de

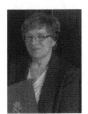

Władysława Pilecka is professor and head of Health Psychology Unit in the Institute of Psychology at Jagiellonian University. Her research interests focus on psychosocial development of children with developmental and medical problems, especially with chronic somatic disease, and intellectual disability. The main topics of her publications are connected with the development of personality and social competencies in these children, and also with supporting this development: psychostimulation and psychocorrection.
Contact: pilecka@apple.phils.uj.edu.pl

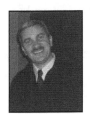

Wojciech Otrębski, professor psychologist, vocational advisor. Head of the Department of Rehabilitation Psychology at the Institute of Psychology, the John Paul II Catholic University of Lublin. Member of the International Advisory Board to *Journal of Intellectual Disability*, UK.
Research interests: rehabilitation psychology, vocational counselling for disabled people, functional diagnosis in rehabilitation psychology, psychological tools for rehabilitation development, early intervention and inclusive education. Scientific consultant to national and international research programmes.
Author, co-author or editor of more than a hundred of publications, e.g. books *Supporting Families With a Disabled Child – Challenges for the Social Services*. Lublin: Europerspektywa, 2011; *I Am an Adult – I Want to Work. Transition From School to Work Training Programme for Youth With Intellectual Disability*. Lublin: Europerspektywa, 2012.
Contact: otrebski@kul.lublin.pl

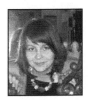

Barbara Czuba, M.A. graduated in psychology at the John Paul II Catholic University of Lublin with specialization in clinical psychology, personality, health and psychotherapy. A child therapist (CBT and SI). She has experience in psychotherapy with children, young people and parents. She provides various forms of psychoeducational classes for children and adults. Her research interests and dissertation concern the operation and assistance to families suffering from allergic disease.
Contact: basia.bartoszek@gmail.com

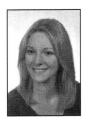

Izabella Januszewska, M.A., Ph.D. student at the Clinical Psychology Department, Institute of Psychology, the John Paul II Catholic University of Lublin, Poland.
The area of interest: coping with stress, clinical health psychology, eating disorders, developmental psychopathology, personality psychology, counselling for patients with hypertension.
Contact: izabellajan@student.kul.lublin.pl

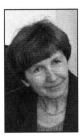

Stanisława Steuden, Ph.D., Full Professor and Head of the Clinical Psychology Department, Institute of Psychology, the John Paul II Catholic University of Lublin, Poland; Chair of the Scientific Council of the Lublin University of the Third Age.
Scientific interests: psychology of aging and old age, burnout syndrome, psychosomatics, diagnosis and counselling for posttraumatic stress disorder, schizophrenia, subjective and objective conditions of resilience and coping with stress.
Contact: stanislawa.steuden@kul.lublin.pl

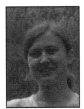

Marta Jurek, M.A. (Pedagogical University of Cracow), Ph.D. student of Jesuit University Ignatianum in Cracow (supervised by Professor Ph.D. Maria Marta Urlińska from Nicolaus Copernicus University in Toruń, Poland), educator (master of pedagogy), child therapist. Her scientific interests: the issues of forming the sense of subjectivity in children and young people, analysis of the context of communication and educational dialogue, pedagogical conditions in developmental and behavioural disorders, problems of rehabilitation of children with disabilities in the social context.
Contact: martaju@autograf.pl

TECHNICAL EDITOR
Dorota Węgierska

PROOFREADER
Monika Zapała

TYPESETTER
Wojciech Wojewoda

Jagiellonian University Press
Editorial Offices: Michałowskiego St. 9/2, 31-126 Kraków
Phone: 12-631-18-80, 12-631-18-82, Fax 12-631-18-83